Survival guide for new parents

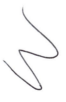

Survival guide for new parents

Pregnancy, birth and the first year

Charlie Wilson

NELL JAMES PUBLISHERS

Published by Nell James Publishers
www.nelljames.co.uk
info@nelljames.co.uk

British Library Cataloguing-in-Publication Data
A catalogue record for this book is available from the British Library.

ISBN 978-0-9567024-5-6

First published 2012.

The Publisher has no responsibility for the persistence or accuracy of URLs for external or any third-party internet websites referred to in this book, and does not guarantee that any content on such websites is, or will remain, accurate or appropriate.

Note: The advice and information included in this book is published in good faith. However, the Publisher and author assume no responsibility or liability for any loss, injury or expense incurred as a result of relying on the information stated. Please check with the relevant persons and authorities regarding any legal and medical issues.

Printed in Great Britain.

To my mummy friends,
without whose honesty and humour this book would not exist:
Angela, Maria, Donna, Donna, Emma and Vicki.
Thank heavens for piling babies on the living room rug
and putting the kettle on.

Contents

Introduction

Welcome! If you've picked up this book it's no doubt because you're expecting, hoping to expect, or have had your first baby. Congratulations – that's great news. You have so much to look forward to in the months ahead. Being a parent is hugely rewarding and so much fun.

But I imagine you already have an inkling that parenting isn't all a bed of roses (well, it is, but the roses aren't de-thorned). Pregnancy, birth and the first year are likely to be the most tiring, difficult and exhausting times in your life – and the most transformative. And that can be a little daunting.

'They should come with a manual' is what most parents of newborn babies say. Well, I don't pretend this book contains everything you could possibly know about babies, but it's a good start. Here, I hope, you'll find out what you need to know to shake off your fears about this journey you're on, to feel good about yourself as a parent and to enjoy the experience.

ABOUT THE AUTHOR

What qualifies me to write a book on being a first-time parent? Well, I'm a mum. I've survived being a first-time parent. And I've talked to a lot of other parents and support organisations while writing this book.

That's it.

I'm not going to try to convince you I'm some kind of 'baby expert'. I've read countless books on parenting (did you know quite a few are written by people who have no kids?), and I've come to the conclusion that there's no such thing as a baby expert. So many people want to tell you how to parent. The truth is, only <u>you</u> know how to parent your baby. You are your baby's mother/father, and only you know how best to be your baby's mother/father. So what you need, rather than do's and don'ts, is some reassuring guidance, advice and support from other parents to help you work out who you want to be as a parent. And that's my aim in this book.

It may interest you to know that I'm far from being a yummy mummy. It took me ten minutes to work out how to do up a sleepsuit the first time I did it. I still do daft things like putting disposable nappies in the washing machine. And I've never quite worked out how to coax my son, George, to let me cut his hair – though I've tried just about every form of bribery there is. A common utterance from my son these days is, 'Oh, silly Mummy.' I don't mind it. I quite like it. George and I have bumbled along together, and along the way we've come up with a way of being together. It works for us. And he's such a happy little boy, I figure I must be doing something right (even if it's not getting him to eat Brussels sprouts).

ABOUT THE BOOK

This book is not meant to be a definitive guide to pregnancy, birth and your baby's first year. Nor is it meant to be stern, bossy and prescriptive. Parenting isn't about rules and hard science: it's about finding out what works for you and your baby. So this book aims to be a gentle and (where appropriate) light-hearted guide to what to expect and how you can be a confident, settled, happy, fulfilled mum or dad (which likely means you have a confident, settled, happy, fulfilled baby).

I've split the book into chapters, each based on a particular theme, and while there is a loose chronology, feel free to read material in any order or to just skip to the chapters that interest you. The book is organised as follows:

- Chapter 1 focuses on parenting styles and covers your instincts, what's important in parenting and being the parent you want to be.
- Chapter 2 focuses on pregnancy and covers the trimesters, medical care, physical symptoms, emotions, baby gear and preparing for parenthood.

• Chapter 3 focuses on birth and covers the last few weeks of pregnancy, birth preparations, labour and birth, tips for dads and handling problems that arise.

• Chapter 4 focuses on the first six weeks and covers the first few days, physical recovery, sleep, basic baby care, visitors and check-ups.

• Chapter 5 focuses on milk feeding and covers being relaxed about feeing, the first feeds, the choice between breast and bottle and how to do each, and feeding routines.

• Chapter 6 focuses on meeting other parents and covers why friends matter, new versus experienced parents, ways to meet other parents, and parent and baby groups.

• Chapter 7 focuses on weaning and covers traditional and baby-led weaning, and how to cope with the mess.

• Chapter 8 focuses on sleep and covers safe sleeping, how babies sleep, sleep deprivation, strategies to improve your baby's sleep, acceptance and alleviating exhaustion.

• Chapter 9 focuses on baby on the move and covers development milestones, the impact of your baby moving about, childproofing and letting your baby explore.

• Chapter 10 focuses on illness and covers instincts, common baby illnesses, when to see a doctor, warding off illness, helping your baby get through illness and coping as a parent.

• Chapter 11 focuses on 'you time' and covers being more than just Mum/Dad, letting go of guilt, thinking back to life before baby and growing as a person.

• Chapter 12 focuses on your partner relationship and covers compromise, communication, couple time and intimacy.

• Chapter 13 focuses on work and childcare and covers dealing with feelings about work, childcare and staying home, choosing who works, flexible working, childcare options and coping at home with your baby.

• Chapter 14 focuses on unexpected issues that can crop up and covers handling feelings about your past, miscarriage,

birth trauma, illness and disability in your baby, post-natal depression and relationship breakdown.
•   And finally, the Useful Resources section points you in the direction of helpful support organisations and websites, and a few films to check out.

Throughout the book, you'll find tips and myth busters, as well as stories from other parents. And because so many of the parents I talked to while writing this book uttered the words 'Why does no one tell you that...?', at the end of each chapter I've compiled some top tips from parents who learned this stuff the hard way.

The easiest approach in writing this book has been to address biological mums and dads, but that isn't meant to exclude single parents or same-sex couples or adopted parents – all the information applies to all kinds of family.

Finally, a quick note on pronouns. I don't like calling a baby 'it' (sounds like a thing, not a person), and the editor in me doesn't like 'they' either (because it's grammatically incorrect). So to solve the issue of pronouns, and in the interests of balance, I alternate between chapters – in chapters with an odd number, pronouns are female; in even chapters, pronouns are male. So apologies if your baby is a boy and you're reading a chapter in which I refer to him as female, and vice versa.

ABOUT THE CHARITY

A third of the royalties of this book go towards Ronald McDonald House Charities. RMHC is a charity that's close to my heart because it helped my family get through a very difficult period.

It is an independent charity that provides free 'home-from-home' accommodation to parents of babies and children in hospital. The charity runs 14 houses beside major children's hospitals in the UK, and 25 family rooms within hospitals, which allow parents to be just a few minutes away from the children's ward at all times. By providing such accommodation, the charity allows families to stay together during the child's illness and have a degree of normality.

My husband and I stayed at RMHC's Camberwell house for several weeks when our son was in King's College Hospital recovering from brain surgery. Before a nurse referred us to RMHC, we were either sleeping one on a camp bed beside George's cot and the other on a chair, or I was staying at the hospital alone with George while my husband commuted back and forth the one-and-a-half-hour journey to our home. Having a room at the RMHC house was a godsend. It enabled both my husband and I to stay with George as he recovered and it meant that while one of us was with George, the other could go back to the house. We took it in turns to have a sleep, have a shower, get some clean clothes and have a meal – all things that are difficult to do in the children's ward. The staff were lovely and so compassionate, and it helped to meet other parents going through the same thing. I look back now and don't know how we would have coped without RMHC.

RMHC is working to raise sufficient funds to develop free accommodation at every specialist children's hospital in the UK. By buying this book, you've helped contribute to this goal. Thank you! I hope you find the book informative, useful and, most of all, reassuring.

1. Being the parent you want to be

If you read just one chapter of this book, I hope it's this one. Because the advice in this chapter can make all the difference to you as a parent.

This chapter lays down the foundations for confident, considered, happy parenting that you can keep in mind throughout the book. The focus is on realising that each parent is different, and that's okay, and that you'll develop confidence in your own style of parenting and in the choices you make.

Forget the rule books full of do's and don'ts for parenting. The truth is that you make your own rules as a parent beyond the basic ones of childcare – and that's what makes parenting fun and rewarding, and that's what your child will grow up to love, respect and admire in you.

TRUSTING YOUR INSTINCTS

Once you have a baby, you know how to parent. You may not think so now, but it's true.

It doesn't matter if you don't know how to do up a nappy. It doesn't matter if you're not sure when babies start eating food. It doesn't matter if you know nothing about baby care at all.

You know how to be a mum or a dad to your baby. And, what's essential to realise is, no one can do it better. You are the best person in the world to be that little person's parent.

The practical stuff you learn along the way (and hopefully this book gives you a helping hand). But the rest, well that's instinct – and you have that already.

Your baby is your baby. You made that baby. She's half you. Only you know what's best for her.

THINKING ABOUT WHAT'S IMPORTANT IN PARENTING

Psychologists have found that the first year of a baby's life is essential to the development of a person. What you do with your baby in year one shapes the person she grows up to be.

That sounds daunting – like you have a massive responsibility and every tiny action and choice you make affects your baby's wellbeing right through her life. Don't worry! There are actually only three things your baby needs from you:

• *Acceptance*. This comes into its own more as your baby grows up and you see a unique personality forming, but from birth you need to accept your baby as she is – a person in her own right with her own feelings and thoughts and desires. You guide her along the way as she grows, but you also let her be who she is. Acceptance goes hand in hand with respect – respect your child and she'll grow to respect you.

• *Attention*. It's said that the greatest gift you can give your child is time. That doesn't have to mean copious amounts of time; for example if you're a working parent you can't necessarily spend as much time with your baby as you'd like. But it means dedicating time regularly to really engage with your baby – so not just cooking dinner while your baby plays nearby under the play gym, but actually playing with your baby, or talking to her, or singing to her, or reading to her and so on. Nothing makes your baby happier than time with Mum and Dad.

• *Love*. All anyone wants is to be loved – it's the most basic human need. So when you're worrying about how well you're doing as a parent, ask yourself: is your baby loved? Does your baby feel loved? Do you kiss her, stroke her head, rub her back, cuddle her often? Do you smile back at her when she smiles at you?

When your baby grows up and looks back on her childhood, what she'll remember are the times you laughed together, the times you played with her, the times you were loving, the times you were proud of her. That's what really matters.

'The most important things – feed my children's minds and souls with good and positive ideas. Teach them morals and ethics. Help them to love learning. Keep their bodies healthy with balanced diets. Provide emotional support whenever needed. Build confidence.'
John, dad to Emile and Gabriel

CONSIDERING THE KIND OF PARENT YOU WANT TO BE
You develop your own style as a parent, and although it hopefully complements your partner's, it is a unique style. You don't sit down one day and decide how you'll parent: you develop your own way over time.

You may be a firm parent or a permissive one. You may be one who loves structure, or one who likes to go with the flow. You may want to teach your baby things, or you may want your baby to learn for herself. You may be an energetic 'Come on, let's go to the park' kind of parent, or you may be one who prefers to potter about at home. You may thrive on mess and chaos, or you may hate the idea of play dough and painting. And so on and so on.

Here are some questions to consider that can help you determine the kind of parent you want to be:
• *Childhood*: What did you like about your childhood? What didn't you? What do you think your parent(s) did right, and what do you not want to do with your child?
• *Education*: What do you want your child to learn about the world, and how?
• *Emotion*: Do you want your child to be free to express how she feels? How will you handle your own feelings?
• *Fun*: What's your idea of fun? How do you intend to enjoy time with your baby? What fun things can you do together? Are you ready to also do what your baby finds fun (even if it's 15 minutes of peek-a-boo)?
• *Lifestyle*: Do you fit around your baby or do you expect your baby to fit around your life? Or a mixture of both? Are

there aspects of your life 'before baby' you want to continue; for example watching footie with your mates or going to the gym? How does your baby fit with these?

• *Mistakes*: How will you handle mistakes, your own and your baby's?

• *Teaching right from wrong*: Little babies don't need to be told right from wrong. But what happens when your nine-month-old keeps throwing her porridge in your face and laughing? And beyond, when Junior's scribbling on the walls in crayon or giving the toilet roll the Andrex puppy treatment?

Parenting is an opportunity to share what you think is good about yourself and the world, and to leave out the stuff you don't like. Hated polishing your shoes as a kid? Detested being made to eat peas and broccoli? Loathed saying grace before a meal? While you hopefully respect why your parent(s) brought you up as they did, this is your chance to rebel and do with your child as you like (and she'll grow up to reject some of the stuff you did in turn!).

IF ONLY SOMEONE HAD TOLD ME: ADVICE FROM PARENTS

• Everyone has an opinion about parenting, and everyone thinks they're right. Perfect the 'I really am listening' smile whilst backing away!

• Whatever rule book you're reading on parenting, your baby hasn't read it. She doesn't know she's meant to nap at half past one for an hour. She's quite content staring at the ceiling and kicking her legs, thank you very much.

• If you've cuddled and smiled at your baby today, you've done well as a parent. Never mind that it took five coffees to get up (and even then you didn't get out of your pyjamas all day).

• Found a strand of spaghetti in your hair? So that's why the bloke in the corner shop was looking at you strangely earlier. Doesn't matter. As long as your baby had fun chucking it there and you laughed together.

- Spending time with your baby is addictive. It's a lot more fun than doing boring jobs around the house. So what if you've a Leaning Tower of Pisa thing going on with dishes in the kitchen sink?

2. Coping with pregnancy

Perhaps you've been feeling a bit strange recently – emotional, off your food, tired, achy in your breasts. Maybe your period is late, when it never is. Or perhaps you've been counting the days until you could open the medicine cabinet and rip open a test.

However you come to the point when you're squatting over a toilet attempting to wee on a little white stick (or waiting patiently outside for your partner to do so), this is a seminal moment. Just one little line, or word, on the test stick will change the course of your life forever. It's a huge, heart-thumping moment.

And there it is: the result. Pregnant.

There may be shouts of joy, there may be beaming smiles, there may be stunned silence. But however you feel as you first discover that you're to become a parent, you can bet that you'll feel this and a whole lot more besides in the coming months.

Pregnancy is a journey – wonderful, exciting, scary, thrilling, fulfilling and exhausting in equal measure. In this chapter, I take you though pregnancy, from that first discovery that there's a tiny person growing inside to preparing the way for your bundle of joy, and help you know what to expect along the way.

GROWING THROUGH THREE TRIMESTERS

A pregnancy lasts just over nine months: 40 weeks in total. Of course, this is just an average. Some women deliver early, some go over their due date. Doctors generally split the 40-week pregnancy into three trimesters as follows:

First trimester: to 12 weeks

A pregnancy is counted from the first day of the last menstrual period, and you're unlikely to know that you're pregnant until a couple of weeks after you conceived. So, on the day you discover you're expecting a baby, you're likely to be between four and seven weeks pregnant already. The first trimester of pregnancy lasts until week 12, so the good news is, you're already halfway there!

During the first trimester, your baby grows from a microscopic speck right after conception to a fully formed baby by week 12 measuring around six centimetres from crown to rump, with fingers and toes and hair and nails. Amazing!

Tip for mums: Make an appointment to see your GP or midwife as soon as you know you're pregnant, so that you can have a check-up and get a scan booked in.

Second trimester: 13 to 28 weeks

Most women find the middle trimester the easiest of the three. Usually, hormones settle, morning sickness disappears and energy levels return to normal. This is an exciting time as Mum's tum grows and grows. Best of all, between weeks 16 to 20 Mum starts to feel the baby wriggling about.

By the end of the second trimester, your baby measures around 24 centimetres from crown to rump and weighs as much as a bag of sugar. By now your baby's eyes are opening, and a thumb-sucking habit may already be established! A baby born prematurely towards the end of this trimester (after week 25) has a chance of survival; every week that goes by from this point onwards, the better your baby's chances.

Third trimester: 28 to 40 weeks

The final rundown to meeting your baby. Mum gets bigger and more tired, and your baby gets more cramped. Watching the skin on Mum's tummy ripple and stretch is mind-boggling as the baby pokes out knees and elbows, and hands and feet.

From week 37, the baby is considered full term, which means it's fine for Mum to go into labour from this point on. Most women deliver at around week 40, though some go over by a week or so – and late babies are common for first-time mums (the term 'late' here always makes me smile; as if babies have a calendar in there and count down to the 'right' day!).

By week 40, your baby measures around 38 centimetres from crown to rump and is a beautiful little creature who's ready to come into the world.

KNOWING WHAT MEDICAL CARE TO EXPECT

Here's a rundown of what to expect from the NHS (assuming you're not going private) from your first appointment to birth:

• *Midwife appointments*: Between eight to 12 weeks you see the midwife for the first time. She asks questions about medical history and lifestyle, and determines your due date. She may take your blood pressure, take blood, test your urine and weigh you. She sees you regularly from that point on, with increasing frequency as you near the birth (most first-time mums see the midwife ten times over the course of the pregnancy).

• *Consultant appointments*: If there are any concerns about Mum or the baby, the midwife will refer Mum to a consultant at the hospital, who makes decisions about care.

• *First ultrasound scan (dating)*: A moment to treasure – when you see your baby for the first time. This usually takes place between eight to 14 weeks. The sonographer checks the pregnancy is viable, checks the baby is developing normally and measures the baby to check the due date is accurate.

• *Second ultrasound scan (anomaly)*: Takes place between 18 and 22 weeks and checks for abnormalities in the baby. You may be able to find out the sex at this scan.

Tip: Don't be afraid to ask questions, and if you're unhappy with an element of your care, say so and/or ask to be transferred to another medical professional.

'The first time I saw Daniel on the screen I cried and cried. I'd had no symptoms of the pregnancy and I think I'd half-convinced myself it was all a dream, not real. But when the guy doing the scan put the wand thing on my

stomach, I heard his heart beating straight away, and then there he was. I couldn't believe how big he was – he looked like a baby. He was dancing about and waving his hands, and it seemed mad that I couldn't feel any of it at all. Then Daniel fell asleep right as the scanning guy was trying to measure something, and he kept jiggling my tummy (my boyfriend was cracking up), and then he asked me to get up and jump up and down a bit. I felt a right idiot! But when I lay back down, he had moved and we could see his tiny little nose and he looked like he was blowing bubbles. We got a picture of that view, and we've kept it on the fridge ever since. That first scan was so great, and I think it was then it really sank in that I was going to be a mummy.'
Janet, mum to Daniel

'I felt excited about the scan and some nervous anticipation, but not worried because I was confident everything would be okay. It made me feel very proud when I saw the baby on the screen and made me look forward to the arrival even more. The only time I've actually thought "Aaargh, my God!" was when my wife first told me she was pregnant (via email!).'
Peter, expectant dad

'I was an emotional wreck before the scan! I was almost in tears in the waiting room and hugely nervous. The relief when we saw the baby wriggling on the screen was overwhelming and I did cry. I hadn't realised how much the stress of waiting for the scan had got to me. I was amazed to see the baby wriggling around and I just so relieved that it was all okay. I felt like I had a weight lifted off my shoulders when we came out and it allowed me to become properly excited about the fact that we're having a baby.'
Wenna, expectant mum

HANDLING THE PHYSICAL SYMPTOMS
It's astonishing how such a tiny being growing in a woman's body can induce such transformations and physical reactions. The human body is a clever machine (though you may doubt its wisdom when it craves a bowl of ice-cream with pickles), and watching Mum grow from lady to baby powerhouse is awe-inspiring. Mum may not feel it at the time, but pregnant women are beautiful – nature at its most miraculous.

Some lucky women breeze through pregnancy feeling on top of the world; others have a miserable time of it, I'm afraid. Nothing can predict how Mum's body will respond to pregnancy and in fact each pregnancy is totally different – you might crawl through your first pregnancy and sail through your second.

Remember, mums, that pregnancy is a temporary, not permanent state, and however you feel, it will pass. Yes, one day you will again leap out of bed without getting a mammoth head rush; you will smell coffee without feeling sick; you will be able to run down a road without waddling like a penguin; you will be able to see your feet!

And if you're concerned about a physical change or symptom, go ahead and speak to your GP or midwife. You're not wasting their time – their job is to check that you're fine and then reassure you of the fact.

Knowing what changes to expect in the body

A woman's body adapts for pregnancy. Mum may notice the following changes:

- *Acne*: Glands often secrete more oil in pregnancy. This can mean dry skin improves (my eczema disappeared while I was pregnant) but it may also mean the occasional juicy pimple.
- *Arched back*: The pelvis tilts and the back arches to help you balance as your bump grows. The back arch can ache.
- *Bigger feet*: Strange but true, your shoe size may increase by half a size or more during pregnancy, as the greater body weight spreads your feet slightly more.

•   *Darkening areolas*: The areola (the area around the nipple) darkens and may enlarge during a first pregnancy.

•   *Different gait*: As you gain weight, your walk changes to adapt to the weight of the baby (fans of the US show *Bones* may remember Temperance Brennan working out a woman was in the early stages of pregnancy just from her gait).

•   *Fast-growing nails*: Don't panic; I'm not talking freaky werewolf claws sprouting overnight. But you may notice you're filing your nails a little more often.

•   *Larger breasts*: You may go up a cup size or two during the pregnancy (and this increase may remain even after you give birth).

•   *Slower pace*: The bigger you get, the slower you move! Infuriated partners may even take to pushing expectant mums uphill.

•   *Stretch marks*: As your breasts and bump grow at a fast rate, your skin sometimes struggles to keep pace and red streaks called 'stretch marks' can appear. There's really not much you can do to prevent these (rubbing moisturiser on may help to give the skin more elasticity). Remember, the red soon fades to a light silver, and these marks bear testament to the fact that your body is carrying your child, so they're something to wear with pride.

•   *Thicker hair*: You lose less hair when you're pregnant due to higher levels of oestrogen and the result is thicker hair. Some women also find their hair is glossier during pregnancy.

•   *Weight gain*: This varies from woman to woman. You gain weight due to the baby, the placenta, the extra blood in your body, the amniotic fluid, and yes, a little extra fat your body puts in reserve, a kind of 'in-case-of-emergency' back-up. After you give birth, much of this weight comes off in the first weeks as long as you eat sensibly during your pregnancy.

Dealing with pregnancy side-effects

You're watching your favourite soap. One of the female characters pushes away her breakfast bowl: 'Feel a bit off it,' she says.

Later that morning, she's having a cuppa in the local caff and complaining to a friend that she's put on weight, when she smells bacon frying and has to run for the toilet. Later still, while arguing with her boyfriend, she hits the deck in a melodramatic faint. Your verdict: she's pregnant.

Ah, the subtlety of the soap world. Most people are familiar with some of the symptoms women can get while pregnant, but there are plenty more you may not be aware of. The following sections look at some of the common physical effects that expectant mums may encounter.

Appetite and taste changes
Women commonly find their eating changes during pregnancy. Food you've always liked becomes repulsive; food you never usually eat becomes delicious. One day you don't feel like eating much at all; the next hubbie comes home to an empty, echoing fridge and a smiling, satisfied wife. It's a weird rollercoaster, but rather good fun if you're willing to ride it.

I remember one shopping trip to the supermarket during my second trimester, and having a nice mooch about, just popping anything I fancied in the trolley. It was only when I was loading the food up on the checkout conveyer belt that I realised the common theme. Bananas, honeydew melon, lemons, cheese, mashed potato, vanilla yoghurt, custard... my body was craving yellow foods. I have no idea why, though a friend who's into colour therapy had quite a lot to say on the matter!

The point is, mad as it seemed, I went with my body. And that's really the best Mum can do. Trust your body, and it'll take care of you and your baby. (And remember that you're less likely to gain a whole heap of excess weight during pregnancy if you eat according to your body's signals.) So if it's a jam and ham sandwich you're craving, give it a go, I say.

Back ache
As I explain in the earlier section 'Knowing what changes to expect in the body', a woman's posture changes during pregnancy

rches. The bigger the bump, the bigger the weight
upporting, and the more likely you'll ache sometimes.

This is a chance for Dad or a friend to give a nice massage or
you can try stretching out with a yoga ball.

Dizziness
It's common to get lightheaded from time to time. Dizziness can
be caused by the lower blood pressure you have during pregnancy, the pressure your womb puts on blood vessels, low blood
sugar or anaemia. Falling over isn't ideal (you may injure yourself
and the baby), so if you feel dizzy, sit down at once and have a
rest, a drink and snack.

Frequent urge to pee
Ah, a delightful side-effect, usually experienced most in the first
and third trimesters. Your womb presses down on your bladder,
leading to a strong urge to pee. Sometimes you'll hot-foot it to
the toilet to find only a dribble emerges. Sometimes the urge will
arrive with shocking suddenness as the baby moves and presses
on the bladder. Sometimes you'll visit the toilet many times in the
course of a day or night.

Tip: If Mum sleeps on the side of the bed that's furthest from
the door, swap sides. The shorter the route to the toilet, the less
the disturbance in the night.

Myth buster: Contrary to popular belief, a policeman/woman
is not going to be impressed if Mum has a pee in his/her helmet.
Pregnant women do get cut some slack, however – if you're
desperate for the toilet while out and about, shops and businesses
should let you use their facilities – but I wouldn't advise extend-
ing the leniency to police attire!

Heartburn and indigestion
Harmless but uncomfortable. Acid reflux caused by hormone
changes and the baby pushing your stomach upwards leads to a
burning feeling in your chest. Eating large meals and lying flat are

key culprits for exacerbating the condition. If you're suffering, look at what you're eating, and how much; try sitting and sleeping propped up; and sip a glass of milk.

Leg cramps

My poor husband. One minute he's sleeping peacefully, the next he's ripped from a happy dream by an ungodly shrieking. Jerking upright, he's prepared for anything: an intruder, a fire alarm, a rampant baboon loose in the house. Instead, he's greeted by me rolling about gripping my calf, which has, out of nowhere, knotted up in a ghastly cramp.

Leg cramps – usually in the calf – are common in pregnancy. Experts don't agree on the cause. Thankfully, the pain eases in a minute or two if you stretch out, massage the muscle or walk it off.

Morning sickness

Morning sickness is a term that covers anything from feeling sick through to actually being sick. Some women end up bent over the toilet; others feel sick a lot, but never get that far. 'Morning' can be quite a misnomer – you may find that nausea comes on later in the day. Some women don't experience any nausea during pregnancy; some women really suffer.

'We've been lucky in that my wife has only felt sick and not actually been sick. I found that the best way to deal with it was to offer support or ask if there was anything she wanted but try not to fixate on the issue or push certain foods/things to do. Accommodate any random requirements but don't be surprised if something she fancies one day is still in the fridge uneaten the next! Don't change habits or wrap her in cotton wool – I didn't treat her any differently to normal.'
Peter, expectant dad

Remember this scene in *Friends*?
>*Phoebe*: Being pregnant is tough on your tummy.
>*Joey*: Hey, but at least you got that cool, pregnant lady glow.
>*Phoebe*: That's sweat. You throw up all morning, you'll have that glow too.

Morning sickness makes you feel far from blooming and radiant, but for the vast majority of women it lasts for a few weeks at most, then you're back to enjoying your food again and travelling without a sick bag in your handbag.

Sleep disturbance

Pregnant women often report waking more in the night, and having vivid dreams. This is likely to be connected to the emotional adjustments of being pregnant, which I discuss in the later section 'Holy cow, we're having a baby: dealing with emotions'.

Stress incontinence

It's a nuisance, it's embarrassing – but it's a fact of pregnancy for many women. Your pelvic floor muscles are the ones that control when you empty your bladder and bowel. During pregnancy, hormones cause your pelvic floor muscles to stretch, which means when you cough or sneeze or jump on a trampoline (!) sometimes a little bit of wee can leak out. The only solution is pelvic floor exercises, lots of them, and often.

When you do a pelvic floor exercise, you basically squeeze muscles down there. The more you use these muscles, you more you strengthen them and the less you leak. And as a bonus, strong pelvic floor muscles are said to shorten the pushing stage of labour. And some people also reckon that pelvic floor muscles improve ability to orgasm. So, worth doing indeed.

To do a pelvic squeeze, imagine that you're trying to stop peeing mid-stream. Easy, right? Yep, but now try again without pulling in your tummy or clenching your buttocks. Ah, now you see. It's a funny sensation. Squeeze down below as you breathe in to a slow count of five, hold for five, and then slowly relax. Build up to repeating the exercise eight times, three times a day. It sounds a lot, but once you get the hang of pelvic floor exercises, you can do them anywhere, anytime – waiting for the kettle to boil, on the bus, during *Coronation Street*.

Sore breasts

Just when Dad's all excited about Mum's expanding bosom, Mum's ready to bash anyone who comes within ten paces of her aching chest. Sometimes breasts are sore, sometimes they're okay. When you think that they're preparing to feed a child, it's fair enough really that they're a little sensitive at times.

Tip: Wearing a good, supportive bra helps ease the soreness, so grit your teeth and get measured by a professional.

Spotting

Light bleeding can occur in healthy pregnancies that go through to term and produce a perfect baby. So the first thing to do if you notice red or brownish discharge is not to panic. Spotting usually stops on its own, but in all cases it's best to call your midwife or GP. They're likely to examine you and may do some routine tests.

Looking after Mum

Watch a visibly pregnant woman enter a room. Everyone in the room looks her way; many smile. People hover anxiously – is she okay? Does she need anything? Does she want to sit down? Humans have an innate impulse to protect and care for pregnant women; after all, we're programmed with this instinct at a primitive level because they're carrying the next generation, securing the continuation of the species.

Being pregnant is perhaps the one time in Mum's life she gets to pull back, take it easy, really look after herself. And it's in looking after Mum that Dad can really get involved with the pregnancy.

Rest

Rest comes first in this section for a good reason: it's essential! Pregnancy is exhausting, and Mum needs more rest than usual. Lots of breaks in the day and early nights are in order.

Stress

Happy Mum equals happy baby. Stress is to be avoided, where possible, during pregnancy. That's not to say Dad has to tiptoe around Mum and never say a cross word; but it does mean that circumstances that are known to expose Mum to prolonged stress (for example, Dad wants to go camping in the Himalayas for a summer holiday, but it's Mum's idea of hell) are to be avoided if possible.

Work is a common source of stress, and it may be that Mum needs to look at her work life with her health and wellbeing in mind, and consider ways to reduce pressure.

Physical activity

Being pregnant isn't a disability; it doesn't have to impede day-to-day activities. Exercise is important to keep healthy, so don't become terrified of moving lest you jar Junior in his cocoon. Exercise as you usually do – swimming and walking are good, gentle activities – and don't push yourself so hard that you become breathless.

There are some forms of exercise it's best to avoid once you're pregnant:
- Contact sports, like judo and kickboxing.
- Sports where there's a risk of falling, such as horse riding, skiing and cycling.
- Scuba diving (the baby can't cope with the pressure underwater).

Also, be careful when lifting heavy items. Pregnant women are more susceptible to straining muscles and ligaments. The perfect excuse to sit back and point to where you want things, while others heft about furniture or bags of shopping.

Tip: Consider doing your food shopping online as your pregnancy advances. That way, you don't need to do any lifting at all.

Eating
Myth buster. Sorry to be a downer, but it's a myth that pregnant women are eating for two. In fact, most women don't need to consume any extra calories at all for the first six months of pregnancy, and only around two hundred a day (the equivalent of a banana and a low-fat yoghurt) for the last three months. So although it's fine for Mum to treat herself from time to time (she deserves it), using pregnancy as an excuse to hugely pig out will lead to excess weight after the baby is born.

Although Mum isn't eating for two in the sense that she needs to eat double quantities, she is eating for the baby too in terms of what she eats. If there was ever a time to eat fresh fruit and veg and cut back on your packet-of-choccie-biscuits-a-day habit, this is it.

I was delighted to be pregnant – obviously, because I wanted to be a mum, but also because, after years and years of watching my weight, I saw it as a sign to relax at last and really enjoy my food. I was really excited about all the foods I would eat, but when morning sickness hit at seven weeks, I had a couple of months of not eating much at all apart from ham sandwiches, bananas and porridge.

Then, when I started feeling better, I found my appetite was much bigger than normal, but I was generally fancying pretty healthy food. That was what my partner calls 'The Smoothie Summer', because I got pretty obsessed with hunting out new fruit combinations to blend up with ice and orange juice. I ate a lot of salad too, and pasta with roasted vegetables.

Of course there was cake and crisps and (my favourite) cheesecake as well, but I was surprised to find I wasn't craving as much junk food as usual.

'I gained a fair bit of weight with Dana, and am a bit curvier than I was before I was a mum now, but only just, and I'm pretty happy at this size.'
Pippa, mum to Dana

I'm not a fan of rules in pregnancy and parenting, but there are some it's best to abide by when it comes to food selection and preparation. Food poisoning is particularly dangerous for pregnant women and unborn babies, so keep the kitchen clean and wash fruit and veg thoroughly. Also, avoid the following foods, which can contain food-poisoning bacteria:

• Raw or partially cooked eggs (there go the dunky soldiers, boo!).
• Raw or undercooked meat.
• Raw shellfish.
• Soft cheeses like brie, camembert, Danish blue and gorgonzola, and mouldy cheeses like stilton.
• Unpasteurised milk and products made from it (such as soft goat's cheese).

Also limit your intake of fish that contain high levels of mercury (which can damage your baby's nervous system). Don't eat shark, marlin and swordfish; and eat the following no more than twice a week: tuna, salmon, mackerel, sardines and trout.

Mum may find, as her bump blossoms, that it's harder to eat larger meals (baby's squashing the stomach, leaving less room). Try 'grazing' through the day instead, eating small amounts here and there.

Tip for mums: If you're eating out in a restaurant, order a starter and dessert, or a children's meal. Or ask for some of your meal to be packaged up to take home for later. It's a break from the norm, but in my experience restaurants are very accommodating of the needs of pregnant women.

'When I was pregnant with my first child, Archie, I remember getting really fed up with all the do's and don'ts

around eating and drinking. The government guidelines were fair enough – I could live without pâté on toast and oysters for nine months! – but I had all kinds of people telling me daft things like cheese causes miscarriage and too much yoghurt can lead to Down's Syndrome. It got pretty upsetting, because I was scared to ignore them in case they were right. Then my partner went and Googled all the foods I was worrying about, and I felt much better once I realised I was fine to eat them. So my advice is to check out what people tell you before getting in a flap!'
Sarah, mum to Archie and Tallulah

Drinking

The Government has recently amended its guidance for alcohol consumption in pregnant women from one unit once or twice a week to recommending complete teetotalism. It's up to Mum how she interprets the guidance; many experts say the odd glass of wine is harmless.

I gave up alcohol completely in my pregnancies; but then I'm not a big drinker anyway, so it was no hardship. I recall rather enjoying being clear-headed and well-rested the day after a friend's party while my husband nursed a hangover.

Just keep in mind that when you drink, the alcohol crosses the placenta into the baby's bloodstream. So when Mum drinks, baby drinks.

The other types of drink to consider are those containing caffeine, too much of which can result in a low birth weight for your baby, and can lead to miscarriage. Experts recommend limiting intake to 200 milligrams a day, which is one to two cups of coffee, or around two cups of tea. Ideally, switch to decaf – and remember that there's caffeine in fizzy drinks, energy drinks and chocolate as well.

Smoking

Smoking is really bad news for your baby (and for Mum). The NHS has a range of support available to help you quit; visit http://smokefree.nhs.uk/smoking-and-pregnancy for more information.

Taking vitamins and medications
A healthy diet provides the vitamins and minerals you need, but during pregnancy doctors recommend taking a supplement containing the following:
- *Vitamin D*: For healthy bones and teeth. Take 10 micrograms of Vitamin D each day throughout your pregnancy and if you breastfeed.
- *Folic acid*: Helps prevent neural tube defects, which can cause conditions such as spina bifida. Take 400 micrograms a day – ideally from before you're pregnant and certainly for the first twelve weeks.

Tip: You can buy vitamins specifically marketed at pregnant women that contain the correct amounts. Buy in bulk over the internet to save money!

When you tell your GP that you're pregnant, he or she should check any regular medications you take to ensure they won't harm the baby. Before taking over-the-counter medicines, check with the pharmacist that they're suitable for pregnant women. Also take care to check any herbal and homeopathic remedies are safe. And stick to paracetamol if you need pain relief.

Guidance from a support organisation: Tommy's
Tommy's exists to give every baby the best chance of being born healthy. Based on extensive research, Tommy's has developed a five-point pregnancy plan to help expectant mums to increase their chances of having a healthy baby:
- *Nutrition*: It's essential to eat a healthy, balanced diet with sufficient vitamins and minerals, especially folic acid, Vitamin D and iron.
- *Weight*: A Body Mass Index (BMI) of 30 or more is associated with a higher risk of pregnancy complications. All

women who are clinically obese are advised to eat a healthy diet during pregnancy and minimise weight gain (dieting in pregnancy is not recommended under any circumstances).

• *Exercise*: Maintain a good level of fitness during pregnancy: at least 30 minutes of moderate, safe exercise every day such as swimming or walking.

• *Smoking*: Seek help from your midwife to give up smoking as soon as possible.

• *Mental health*: If you're struggling emotionally, and suffering from anxiety and depression, tell your midwife or GP so that you're put in touch with the appropriate services or support groups.

For further pregnancy information, call Tommy's specially trained midwives on 0800 0147 800 or email info@tommys.org. To order your guide to healthy pregnancy, visit www.tommys.org.

HOLY COW, WE'RE HAVING A BABY: DEALING WITH EMOTIONS

Having a baby is a big deal. Nothing creates such a vast scale of emotion, from creeping fear and anxiety to rushes of love and joy. The emotional journey can be a bit overwhelming, but if you can sit with the feelings and accept them as totally normal, you soon feel more settled and in control of your emotions. I can't promise, though, that you'll ever watch poorly babies on *Comic Relief* appeals again without becoming a basket case.

Riding the mood swings

Ah, the rollercoaster of pregnancy. One minute Mum's laughing and singing and dancing around the kitchen; the next she's sobbing into the sofa cushion. One day Dad is day-dreaming about playing footie in the park someday with his kid; the next he's watching a toddler have a tantrum in the supermarket and feeling hot and sweaty at the thought of having one of those to contend with.

Mum can blame hormones as much as she likes (and of course they play a part in the emotional ups and downs), but the truth is that both Mum and Dad encounter varying moods during pregnancy. There's so much to get your head around, and that has an impact on your emotions.

The best you can do is ride the highs and stumble through the lows, knowing that soon enough you'll feel better, more in balance again. And be kind to each other.

Wrestling with 'baby brain'

Pregnant women often report finding it harder to focus and concentrate, and having foggy and absentminded periods. You may find your car keys in the fridge. You may totally forget your sister's birthday. You may order a coffee in your local cafe, pay and then walk out without the drink.

Don't panic if it happens to you – you're not losing your mind, you simply have a touch of baby brain. Laugh it off and have a break and you'll soon feel better.

Becoming fascinated by babies and parents

You find out you're pregnant, and suddenly there are babies everywhere! You go to a public place and there they are – in their buggies, on mums' laps, on dads' shoulders, screaming, crying, laughing, gurgling, waving their fat little fists in the air. Baby overload!

Of course, you've always been surrounded by babies, but now you've one on the way, you're more attuned to noticing them. You find yourself watching, fascinated. You stare at bumps on pregnant ladies. You peer in passing buggies to check out the snoozing occupant. You pull silly faces at a baby across a restaurant.

You wonder what your baby will be like in comparison; how you'll parent in comparison. You worry that you won't know how to soothe your baby like that woman does. You fret that your baby won't be a cute as that one. You wonder whether you'll be as chilled as that dad looks. You look around at other parents and they seem so confident, so in control; like they know what they're doing. But they were once in your shoes – they've learnt how to look after baby, just as you will.

Becoming more interested in babies and parents around you is a normal part of the emotional adjustment to becoming a mum or dad. Observing others helps you pick and choose what you like and don't like in parenting styles (more on this in Chapter 1), and it helps you gain confidence that there's a whole world of people out there bringing up kids. Yes, having a baby is a big deal, but many, many people do it. They get through the hard stuff and enjoy the good stuff. You're not alone.

Accepting Mum's changing body

In the earlier section 'Knowing what changes to expect in the body', I outline some of the ways in which Mum's body changes during pregnancy.

Women react differently to the pregnant form. Some women adore pregnancy, especially the big bump; others struggle with their feelings. Here are feelings that pregnant women can develop:

•   *Feeling fat*: What woman finds it easy, in today's society, to gain weight? Many women report feeling relieved once their bump becomes obvious, because then its apparent to the world they're pregnant, not just carrying some extra weight on the tum. The weight you gain will come off again after birth with healthy eating and some light exercise; for now, the baby needs this weight for its cosy cocoon.

•   *Feeling ugly*: Okay, swollen ankles, varicose veins, zits and stretch marks aren't sexy, but in time they'll diminish.

'I suffered from an eating disorder in my teens. Although I'm better now, I'm still sensitive about my weight, so I was really worried about how I'd handle the weight gain when I was pregnant. And I was anxious that whatever weight I put on I'd struggle to lose afterwards. But actually, as I got bigger, I found it quite exciting rather than

upsetting. I measured my bump each week and put the numbers into a spreadsheet to make a graph – sad, I know, but I loved it! I think because the bump is so hard, it didn't feel like fat to me. After I gave birth I didn't like the soft tummy I had left, but in a few months I was back to my usual shape pretty much.'
Pippa, mum to Matthew

'Many women complain about the changes in their body during pregnancy. However, after many years of fluctuating between reasonable healthy weight and 'a tad on the hefty side', I actually felt it was quite liberating being pregnant as there was no longer any pressure to maintain a slender frame. My additional pregnancy weight was looked on favourably by family, friends and strangers alike, with positive comments about my lovely child-bearing hips and bountiful breasts, perfect for rearing healthy children. I have never been so complimented. In fact, I even chose to have semi-clothed professional bump photography done and was very pleased with the outcome.'
Frances, mum to Erin and Olivia

Here are some tips for mums feeling unhappy in their skin:
•	Ask your partner or a friend (or a professional photographer) to take some photos of you with your bump. You may be surprised how much you like the look of yourself in the photos. And they're great to keep for posterity – post-pregnancy you'll be amazed at the size of the bump!
•	Buy maternity clothes in which you feel comfortable and attractive.
•	Indulge yourself in some pampering treatments while pregnant to really take care of your body.
•	Talk to other pregnant ladies, if you know any, about how they feel, and talk to mums. You'll find reassurance that your worries are common, and that in time you'll feel better about how you look.

- Take time each day to sit with the baby – feel the baby under the skin of your bump, moving about. Your bump isn't a huge mass of fat; there's a beautiful baby curled up in there!

Dads also have feelings about their partner's body as it changes. Some men find the changes of pregnancy beautiful, and fancy their partner more by the day. They look at the growing bump and are simply blown away by the notion that their son or daughter is inside. Others are a little taken aback by the rapid expansion of the woman they love. Here are some tips for dads:

- It's okay not to love your partner's new shape, but please don't tell her if this is how you feel! Your job, as her partner, is to support her, and women are notoriously sensitive about their looks.
- Compliment your partner regularly – be genuine, though; she'll see through blatant lies ('You're as slim as the day I met you, love') or random comments ('That maternity smock is lovely; you should keep that to wear after the baby's born').
- Treat your partner to massages – the bump, her back, her feet. It's a lovely way to relax her and make her feel that her body is beautiful to you.

Feeling randy, or anything but

Some couples find they get closer during pregnancy, and Mum, in particular, may have an awesome hormone high that induces lustful episodes. If you find pregnancy ramps up your sex life, great, go with it. You may have to adapt positions as Mum grows, but as long as you're not attempting anything too ambitious and strenuous (remember, pregnant women aren't that bendy …) your baby will be fine.

Equally, however, Mum or Dad (or Mum and Dad) may go right off sex during pregnancy. Some mums are just too tired, or emotional, or sore. Some dads struggle to see the pregnant form as sensual. And some parents feel uncomfortable about the proximity of the baby to, ahem, Dad's appendage. One friend told me she had an awful vision of the baby seeing what was going on (anatomically impossible, of course), and that was the end of bedroom games until after the birth.

If sex becomes difficult or uncomfortable for you, don't worry about it. You can soon get back on track after your baby's born, and in the meantime there's a whole host of things you can do with your partner to demonstrate love and affection – whether it's sexual acts that don't lead to penetration, or simply massages, cuddles, kisses and so on.

A final note on dreams. Most pregnant women I know admit to having some pretty racy dreams. Don't panic: just because you dreamed about doing unspeakable things to the plumber who cleaned out your drains, or the bloke who runs the local fish-nibbling-at-your-feet spa, or that uber-geek from *The Big Bang Theory*, doesn't mean you actually want to pounce on said man, or that you're being unfaithful to your partner. It's just a dream. Just hormones.

Managing anxiety

Pregnancy can be an anxious time. Not only do you have your feelings about whether you'll be a good mum or dad to contend with (trust me, the very fact that you're worrying about this shows that you care, so of course you will be), but you worry about whether baby will be okay. Babies are so tiny and fragile, and you can easily drive yourself mad thinking about everything that could potentially go wrong during pregnancy.

Two thoughts for you: thinking positive never hurts, and worrying never achieves anything. As long as Mum's being sensible and taking care of herself then there's nothing more you can do to protect your baby. As hard as it is, you can't control how the baby grows and develops – you just have to do your best to have faith and relax.

Another source of anxiety may be Mum's health. This was certainly something I struggled with while pregnant, as my own mother died young, just days after having me. But again, worrying gets you nowhere. If there are health issues, let the consultant at the hospital take charge. Otherwise, remind yourself that you're in the 21st century, and medical care and technology these days are excellent.

> 'I had awful nightmares when I was pregnant – about losing the baby, about the birth and about being a mum. In one I gave birth to an ostrich! It all seems silly now, but at the time I was so emotional and scared, and the dreams were so real and vivid. My advice if you're worrying at night is to get up, turn on the light, go make a hot drink and watch some tele to distract yourself. In the light of day in the morning, you'll feel much calmer.'
> Lana, mum to Max

Understanding and coping with negative feelings

Pregnancy is supposed to be a wonderful blessing, months of wonder and happiness in a woman's life, right? Well, no, not necessarily. It's something of a taboo subject, but the truth is that many women struggle with negative feelings about their pregnancy.

The 2007 film *Waitress* – which is about a pregnant, unhappily married waitress called Jenna who's having an affair with her doctor, Jim – touches upon this subject. Jim tells Jenna that she's beautiful. Jenna disagrees, and tells him she's fat. Jim tells Jenna that she's not fat, she's pregnant, and there's nothing more beautiful than having a baby growing inside you. This is Jenna's response: 'It's an alien and a parasite. It makes me tired and weak. It complicates my whole life. I resent it. I have no idea how to take care of it. I'm the anti-mother.'

At times you may feel and think some of the following:

• *Scared*: Will I be a good mum? Will I enjoy being a mum? Will I cope with giving birth? Just how much will it hurt? What if the baby's ill or damaged in some way? What if the baby's ugly? What if I hate the baby? What if I don't love him? What if I do something stupid like drop the baby on his head?

- *Resentful*: This baby is taking over my body – it's making me feel ill, it's making me ugly (stretch marks, weight gain and so on), it's making me tired and slow. This baby is getting in the way of things I want to do – going out with friends, having a few drinks, travelling abroad, pushing forward my career. This baby is changing things between me and my partner – my partner loves me less now, is less interested in me. And when it comes, I don't want to be so needed; I want my own space and my own life. I like my life as it is; I don't want it to change!

- *Overwhelmed*: I can't do this! I can't give birth. I'm not strong enough. I can't be a mummy. I don't know what to do. There's so much I don't know – so many things I need to know. It's all too much.

- *Invaded*: There is a person inside me. Euh! The bigger he gets, the less room there is for me. He's pushing at me and kicking at me and my bump feels ready to explode. I don't want company. I want to be alone in my skin! He doesn't feel like a he; he feels like an it.

- *Repulsed*: What is happening to my body! Urgh, my breasts, my thighs, my stomach – huge! My skin, yuck! This massive bump – it's so ugly, repulsive. And then there are the babies. I see them around. I don't get what all the fuss is. They're not that cute. In fact, they look like cross, poopy, noisy little things to me that leach on and demand and demand and demand.

There are a lot of difficult thoughts and feelings there. You may have none of these. You may have some of these once in a while. You may have some of these often. You may have many of these most of the time, and more besides.

In short, you may discover that you really don't like being pregnant at all. And because of your negative feelings, you may worry that you shouldn't be having this baby at all, or that you're going to be a bad mother.

Women who are struggling with being pregnant often feel ashamed of their feelings, because this isn't an aspect of pregnancy often discussed. When you tell people you're pregnant, their automatic response is, 'Wonderful news! Congratulations!', not, 'Oh, poor you. That's going to be a tough few months, hmm?' To anyone outside of the pregnancy, it's miraculous, amazing, fabulously happy. To the woman whose body is expanding rapidly, who's housing another person and who at some point has to push that person out and then care for it, pregnancy is a little less straightforward.

When you find yourself having a difficult thought or feeling, don't feel bad. Every woman gets down or frustrated about being pregnant at some point, some more than others – just think, by 40 weeks even the happiest pregnant lady is desperate for the baby to come out so she has some space to breathe again! There's no rule that pregnancy has to be a walk in the park; pregnancy is whatever you experience it as. And who says morning sickness and tiredness and mood swings and having your organs squashed by a baby have to be fun?

If pregnancy is hard work for you, that's okay. Although it seems it when you're pregnant, it doesn't last forever. (Pity the poor elephant, who carries her baby for 22 months!) Let yourself have the feelings without feeling bad, and reassure yourself that soon it will be over and you'll look back on the pregnancy from a happier place and feel like it passed in a blur. And if you haven't watched the film *Waitress*, give it a go – despite her negative feelings, Jenna becomes a happy mum.

Tip: If your feelings about being pregnant are really upsetting you and affecting your life, have a chat with your midwife or GP. It might be that a short course of counselling will help.

Bonding with your baby
There's a person growing inside Mum. If you think about it, that's pretty amazing, and also perhaps pretty bizarre. Another person inside a person! I remember the first time I showed my best friend Sarah (not a mum yet) George digging out his tiny

elbow in my bump, and she was intrigued by the moving lump under my skin but also honest enough to admit she was kind of freaked out. I think she began a discussion on the film *Aliens*, and I tuned out at that point.

It's a big adjustment to really understand that there's a baby inside Mum, and not just any baby, your baby – half mum and half dad. The whole experience feels so surreal: how does this rounded belly turn into a tiny person with thoughts and feelings and moods?

You may feel pretty comfortable with the idea of becoming a parent, and connected to the growing child. But it's okay not to feel instantly like a mum or dad; not to feel instant adoration for this invisible, intangible baby that you can't see yet.

Once your baby's born, the bond grows. Remember, nothing feels real about pregnancy until you hold your baby in your arms. You will love your child. Your child is yours – yours! – and that feels very different to how you connect to any other human being on the planet.

If you want to do more to connect to your baby in the womb, here are some ideas you can try:

- *Ask for pictures.* Take home photos from your ultrasound scans and look at them often. If your budget can stretch to it, have a private scan and spend some time looking at your baby.
- *Talk/sing to baby.* From around week 21 baby can hear beyond the womb, and studies have found that babies recognise their parents' voices after the birth if they've heard them often enough in the womb.
- *Play your favourite music to the bump.* My husband created a seven-disc 'Bump' compilation to educate George in music pre-birth. Hard work for me at times when we reached a song not to my taste!
- *Buy and/or make things for the baby.* A teddy, a blanket, knitted booties – some little object you buy or make with affection helps you connect.

- *Name baby*. Giving the baby an identity can help with bonding. Some parents choose a generic name – 'Lil' Bean', 'Bumpy', 'Bubbie', 'Peanut' and so on. Then, if you choose to find out the sex, you can later start using the baby's real name (more on choosing a name in the later section 'What's in a name?').
- *Spend time with your baby*. Try to make a little time each day just to be together as a family – a chance for Mum and Dad to watch the baby wiggle about and to talk to the baby. This is especially important for dads, who don't feel the baby moving all day long like mums do.

DISCOVERING YOU'RE HAVING MORE THAN ONE BABY

Multiple births are increasingly common now that more couples are using IVF to help them conceive.

Some people are delighted at the thought of having more than one baby at a time. You may be thinking:
- Hooray! The more the merrier.
- A readymade family.
- I only want two kids, so twins means I get all the hard work of the early years out of the way at once.

Some people are a little less enthralled. You may be thinking:
- Oh cripes! How can we afford/fit in/look after an extra child/children?
- It'll be total chaos. How will we cope?
- I'll never get my figure back.
- I wanted to focus all my attention and love on one for now; will my children get less of me?

Many people will feel the two extremes of emotions at once: joy and fear. That's okay; that's normal. It's a shock to discover not an extra person (or two, or three) hanging out in Mum's tum – give yourself some time to adjust to the idea.

Then, once you've got used to the idea, check out what support is available to you. In most areas your midwife can put you in touch with a multiple birth group, where you can meet other mums and dads with twins and triplets (and perhaps even more). And the organisation TAMBA (Twins and Multiple Births Association; www.tamba.org.uk) offers all kinds of support, including a helpline and a forum.

'On the way up to the hospital to have a scan at eight weeks we knew we would find out whether we were expecting one or two babies (we'd had IVF, and they had put two embryos in). On the way up Greig said he thought he would be disappointed if it was only a singleton... phew! I knew I was having twins. Well, did I really know or do I just say that? I had been feeling sick almost since the day they implanted the embryos, and the pregnancy test line was instant and very strong. Anyway the sonographer asked that we give her some time to scan and then she would tell us what she could see. She began the scan and shortly after raised her eyebrow. Greig and I looked at each other and we knew...twins. My tips for parents of twins? Try not to compare yourself with single parents (what we call parents with a single, not multiple, birth). It is completely different. And do whatever works for you!'
Alison, mum to Hannah and Emily

'For me I knew there was a chance we could be having twins. No matter how much you might prepare yourself it is still a shock when you are told. Two babies! Embrace it, enjoy it and get involved. Don't ask single daddies how much sleep they get...you'll be getting as much as mummies! People say double trouble, but it is double the fun, double the reward and double the love too.'
Greig, dad to Hannah and Emily

GETTING PRACTICAL: BABY PARAPHERNALIA

I know many parents (my husband and myself included) who admit that at some point during the pregnancy they stood in a babyware shop and had a total meltdown. Buggies, car seats, cots, Moses baskets, bouncy chairs, high chairs, baths, play gyms, play mats, sterilisers, breast pumps, monitors, mobiles, lullaby music makers... the sea of baby gadgets threatens to engulf you, and that's before you even look at nappies and wipes and shampoo and clothes – so many clothes! Where do you start? How much do you spend? What do you actually need?

I remember stumbling out of Mothercare gripping a teddy – the one thing I'd managed to buy – and sniffling to myself that I was going to be a terrible mum because I couldn't even work out how to collapse the travel system we'd looked at. I look back now and smile; but at the time I was in an utter panic. And I remember my husband saying, daunted, 'Where are we gonna put all this stuff!', because at the time we lived in a tiny two-bed house.

The truth is, most of the items in a babyware shop are luxuries, not essentials. But such is the range on offer, and the power of the marketing, that new parents struggle to know what to buy.

Here's what you actually need for your new baby:

- A car seat if you have a car.
- A couple of sheets and blankets.
- Bottles and a steriliser if you intend to bottle feed.
- Cotton wool for cleaning.
- Nappies – whether reusable or disposable.
- Something for the baby to sleep in (a cot or a Moses basket – or a drawer worked fine for our great-grandmothers!)
- Something for baby to wear – ten babygros and ten vests will do you for the first weeks (babies grow very fast, remember!), plus a jacket or snowsuit (depending on the season) for going out.
- Something to carry the baby in if you don't want to carry him in your arms all day: a buggy or sling or baby carrier.
- Something for wiping up milky burps – muslin squares (mussies) are ideal: cheap and machine washable.

- Thermometer (ear ones are easiest).

And here are some items you may find useful:
- A packet of dummies (even if you're sure you won't use them, have a pack in case).
- Baby monitor if your house is big enough that you won't hear him cry.
- Colic medicines – ask your pharmacist for advice.
- A dimming lamp you can use to feed your baby by (if you don't have a dimmer on your overhead light) – nothing's worse than a 100-watt bulb blinking on in the dead of night.

Remember that you don't need lots of stuff straight away – things like high chairs and toys can come later (your baby won't be interested in toys until around the sixth week).

'Gadgets – now that's a bit of preparing for a baby I could really get into. Best buy, I think, was a video monitor so we can see what Claire's up to once we put her to bed. It's hilarious sometimes what she does – we put the monitor by the tele and end up watching her more than the TV! At first you're hyper-sensitive to it and notice every little movement, then you relax.'
Adam, dad to Claire

In their excitement about the new baby, and their nesting activities, many new parents splash out, creating a beautiful nursery and putting a lot of time, effort and money into filling their homes with stuff for the baby. If this makes you happy, that's fine, of course. But you don't have to splash the cash if you don't want to (or don't have it to spend!). Here are some ideas for saving money:
- Look forward to gifts! Visitors will flood to see the new baby, and they'll bring baby toys and probably clothes as well. If Grandpa wants to buy a present, you can suggest something

practical (rather than the terrifyingly enormous and entirely useless teddy bear he was planning to buy).

• If you know someone with a baby, ask whether you can borrow some clothes. Little babies get very little wear out of clothes because they grow out of them so fast, so they're good to be reused.

• Use the kitchen sink, instead of a baby bath. Once your baby outgrows the sink, you can lay him flat on the bottom of a very shallow bath (on a bath mat or towel) and he can kick and splash as you wash him.

• Second-hand bargains. Check out your local National Childbirth Trust (NCT) branch to find out when their next nearly new sale is. You'll be amazed what you can pick up at a fraction of the cost you pay in the shops. Also look at local listings sites like Gumtree and your local Netmums board, and on eBay.

PREPARING FOR TWO TO BECOME THREE

Having a baby is huge. It's going to change your life forever (but in a great way, honest!). Once the dust settles after you discover you're pregnant, you have seven months or so to get used to the idea of having another member of the family – indeed, you may even see it as becoming a family, rather than a couple.

You've plenty of time to adjust to the idea, and to decide how your baby will fit into your lives. Chapter 1 explores the kind of parent you'd like to be. But here I take you through some practical considerations to make when your baby goes from being a twinkle in your eye to a reality whose arrival grows closer by the day.

Telling people about the baby

Every couple is different and whenever you choose to tell people that you're pregnant is your choice. Some parents tell the world straight away; some tell only close family until after the first scan;

some wait even longer. You need to do whatever feels right to you.

The reasoning behind waiting to tell people is that, sadly, miscarriage is common in the first weeks. In the second trimester the risk of miscarriage drops by around 65 per cent, and people feel more secure telling the world at that point.

What you need to consider is who, if the unthinkable happened and you lost the baby, you would want to know, and who you'd rather not.

As an example, in my second pregnancy we told close friends and family straight away, and we also told our son (aged two at the time), whom we expected wouldn't remotely take in the news. But actually, George was very excited and proceeded to tell anyone we met – including some neighbours and all the staff at his nursery. When we discovered we had lost the baby, I didn't regret having told close friends and family, because they were a source of support for me. But I could have done without having to explain the loss to the neighbours and my son's nursery staff – they were very nice, of course, but it felt a personal loss that I'd rather not have had to discuss with them.

Tip for mums: You don't have to tell your employer that you're pregnant until the 15th week prior to your baby's due date (so roughly 25 weeks) unless there are health and safety implications for you working while pregnant (for example, your job involves lifting). Think about when will be best to tell your boss; timing will depend on your work situation. And remember, it's illegal for an employer to dismiss or unfairly treat a woman because she's pregnant.

Finding out the sex

Do you or don't you? And if you find out, do you keep it to yourself or tell the world?

Sometimes sonographers conducting the second NHS scan will tell you, if you want to know it, their opinion on what the sex of your baby is. Do bear in mind that this is an opinion – it's not 100 per cent foolproof. On some babies it's obvious, on some it's a little less clear. I have a friend who was told her first baby was a girl, when it was a boy; and that her second was a boy, when it was a girl. She was very glad she'd stuck to fairly neutral clothes and colour schemes in the nursery!

Tip: If you really want to know the sex, a private scan (from 14 weeks) will confirm this for you. They cost from around £90.

'I didn't want to know the baby's sex. I wanted it to be a surprise. But John did want to know. We agreed that we wouldn't ask, because it was important to me. But then, at a dinner party a few weeks later, John was talking about the baby and he said "he". I was furious! Turned out he'd asked the woman doing the scan while I'd gone out of the room to go to the toilet. I was excited to find out we were having a boy, but I missed the surprise.'
Lorna, mum to James

What's in a name? Choosing a name for baby

Most parents will choose a name, or several options for names, during pregnancy. If you find out the sex of the baby, you may even start using that name while baby's still in the womb. Alternatively, you may pick a name for a girl and one for a boy; or you may have a shortlist and decide you'll choose once you meet the baby.

Choosing a name is a fun job during pregnancy, but beware: it can cause disagreement between Mum and Dad! My husband and I found settling on a girl's name easy enough, but when we found out we were having a boy, we struggled to agree. My husband didn't like the names I chose; I couldn't stand his. Finally, one day we descended to messing about and calling out names we'd never pick – Marmaduke, Horacio, Dastardly, Muttley – and then, jokingly, my husband threw George into the mix. And we realised we both loved it.

Here are just a few tips for picking a name:
• Don't choose a name that's shared by an ex-girlfriend or ex-boyfriend unless you want that person to see on Facebook

that you've named your firstborn after him/her, and wonder whether you still hold a torch.

• Think about how the name will fit a baby, a toddler, a child, a teenager and a grown man or woman.

• Consider whether the name will embarrass the child.

• Think about how the name fits with the surname.

'I went through 100,000 names only to arrive at one that I had liked before we even opened the book! Hubbie was yet to be convinced on the name "Ava", and came up with an alternative, "Summer". When she arrived, we knew that she didn't look like a Summer, so by default she became Ava.'
Emma, mum to Ava

Clearing space in your home?

As I explain in the previous section on baby paraphernalia, one of my husband's early concerns was where we were going to put all the baby stuff in our house.

Babies are tiny little creatures when they first arrive, and yes, they come with some gear, but they don't take up that much room – especially when they're newborn. All you need is a little room to play as the baby gets older, and somewhere for him to sleep. He may sleep in with you for keeps; or you may set aside a room to be the nursery.

Tip: If you do decide to set up a nursery, and you want to decorate it, do so a few weeks before baby is due. The room needs time to air so Junior isn't inhaling paint fumes.

Thinking about maternity and paternity leave

Mums and dads are entitled to time off work to spend with their baby.

• Mums can have up to a year off work: 26 weeks Ordinary Maternity Leave, followed by 26 weeks Additional Maternity Leave. Maternity leave can start at any point from the

11th week before the baby is due. You need to check with your employer what pay you're entitled to during this time.

• Dads can take up to two weeks off (in one block) within the eight weeks after the baby is born, and they receive Ordinary Statutory Paternity Pay. They can also opt to take Additional Paternity Leave for up to 26 weeks.

The details of maternity and paternity leave are quite complicated: qualifying for the leave, informing your employer, what pay you receive and so on. Take a look at the Direct.gov (www.direct.gov.uk) website for details.

Of course, neither maternity nor paternity leave lasts forever – at some point, Mum and/or Dad has to go back to work. Who's going to take care of baby during the working week? Chapter 12 looks at work, childcare options and stay-at-home parenting in detail. Before the baby comes, it's a good idea to consider your options.

Taking a babymoon
Happy babies have happy parents, and the more nice couple time Mum and Dad have before the birth, the better. Once the baby arrives, the first weeks are going to be tiring and an adjustment, and you may find your relationship goes on the back burner. Invest some energy into your relationship during pregnancy and you've got some love and affection in reserve for later.

Go on some dates, snuggle up in front of a movie, or, if you've the time and the budget, why not take a 'babymoon' – your last holiday as a childless couple. Even if the most you manage is a night away in a bed and breakfast, the time you spend together is great for grounding you as a couple about to become parents; and you can look back on the memory fondly when you're knee-deep in milky mussies and dirty nappies in the months to come.

For more on focusing on your relationship, check out Chapter 13.

IF ONLY SOMEONE HAD TOLD ME: ADVICE FROM PARENTS

- Add pantiliners, spare knickers, indigestion chews and other non-sexy equipment to lippie, purse, keys, mobile and so on you already lug about.
- While travelling on the tube, a 'Baby on Board' car sticker front and back is a good deterrent for sharp-edged-briefcase-wielding chaps.
- Babies on an ultrasound screen look like aliens (especially on 3D scans). Don't panic. Babies scrub up just fine.
- An outy becomes a pointy; an insy becomes a crator. Belly buttons become fascinating. But don't expect others to be similarly interested.
- Always, always tell a pregnant woman that she looks great. Even if she's got a zit in the middle of her forehead you're struggling not to stare are and is wearing a dress the size of a six-person tent.
- If you're worried your baby hasn't moved for a while, poke him!
- Plan a cutting comeback for the line, 'Look at the size of you!' Something like, 'And look at the size of you!'

3. Meeting your baby: the birth

The day your baby is born is going to be the biggest day of your life so far. How you feel when you first see your child surpasses anything you've felt before. It's an amazing, exciting, wonderful time. And, of course, it's all rather scary, exhausting, painful and messy too!

In this chapter, I take you though those last weeks of pregnancy through to holding your baby in your arms. The point of the chapter is to reassure you that this is a worthwhile experience that you'll look back on with a sense of pride and accomplishment, and to give you confidence in making the right choices for Mum and baby throughout.

COUNTING DOWN: THE LAST FEW WEEKS

The last few weeks of pregnancy are pretty tough. Mum's tired, uncomfortable and totally over the novelty of having a kicking, wriggling baby in her belly. And the impending birth is looming, which can create feelings of fear and anxiety in both parents.

Struggling to sleep

When you're about to become a mum, people advise you to get plenty of sleep before birth and enjoy your lie-ins. But you can't. Because you can't get comfy, you need the toilet once an hour, you're hot and you're soon going to have a baby, which keeps you awake, worrying.

It's normal to find your sleep steadily more disturbed as you approach the birth. You may even decide this is nature's way of preparing you to be a mother of a newborn, who'll wake often at night to start with. If you went from sleeping a solid ten hours a night to being up every couple of hours it would be a terrible shock.

This is the point at which you need to start resting when you can – which, if possible, means resting/napping in the day.

And if you're very pregnant and very sleepless, don't dash about doing jobs at 3 a.m. Try to take it easy, because your insomnia may be a sign of labour on its way (and so you need to conserve your energy). I spent the night before I went into labour with George sitting up watching cheesy made-for-TV films, wondering why I was so alert.

Feeling uncomfortable

Late pregnancy is no picnic. Dad, you might be wondering how Mum could possibly get any bigger; rest assured, she's thinking the same thing. The baby is super squished now, and sometimes her stretching and moving can be pretty uncomfortable for Mum. Plus Mum might have developed some late pregnancy side effects, like swollen feet, an aching back, heartburn and feeling very hot.

Taking it easy is the best remedy for discomfort. Remember, although time may be dragging now, it won't be much longer until Mum gives birth and her body starts to recover.

Coping with your feelings

You may have all kinds of feelings in the last weeks, such as excitement that you're soon going to meet your baby, and anticipation for what lies ahead. But the feelings you're most likely to struggle with are anxiety and fear – will Mum and the baby be okay through the birth?

It's natural to worry, but try to remember that childbirth is a completely natural process, and with modern medicine, the chances are very good that everything will be fine.

Talk about your concerns with each other (a problem shared is a problem halved, as they say), and think about whether there are practical things you could do to ease the anxiety. For example, is Mum worrying about Dad missing the birth? Come up with a plan to ensure this won't happen (and Dad, cancel any trips out of town!). Or is Dad worrying that he'll crumble in the delivery room? Chat to other fathers who can help Dad know what to expect, and perhaps think about having a second person in the delivery room with you, if permitted, as extra support for both Mum and Dad.

Being random

Women who are soon to have a baby can do some quite random things. That's okay; that's normal!

For example, as a pregnant woman approaches her due date, the nesting impulse kicks in, and Mum may go on a cleaning frenzy or insist on rearranging furniture in a room. Dad, just go with it! It's not necessarily a rational impulse at times, but it's totally natural. At least, this is what I told my husband when, three weeks before my son was due, I had him whitewashing the dark, dank cellar (quite what use I thought that was to the baby I've no idea, but it seemed essential at the time!).

> 'I just could not get the kitchen clean enough. I scrubbed and scrubbed. And I washed all the baby clothes twice. And I cooked and cooked. I was glad of it, though, when Joy came because we had a freezer full of meals.'
> Zola, mum to Joy

You may also find that Mum is a bit all over the shop, with see-sawing emotions and the ability to execute a surprising U-turn out of nowhere. This is especially the case when it comes to decisions you've already made about the birth (see the later section 'Preparing for birth') – as Mum approaches delivery, her instincts may direct her to change her mind, and it's important to go with what Mum feels she wants. For example, you may have planned a water birth all through the pregnancy, but suddenly, a few weeks before the due date, Mum decides she doesn't want one at all. Mum knows best!

PREPARING FOR BIRTH

Mum's no doubt been thinking about what you want for baby's birth from the first weeks of pregnancy, and has already discussed a birth plan of sorts with the midwife. The last weeks of pregnancy are the time to firm up your ideas.

Tip: You may write a birth plan during this time, laying down your preferences. It's a good idea, because it helps you determine what you want and communicate that to the medical professionals who'll be looking after you. But don't set it in stone. Be prepared to modify, or totally scrap the birth plan if necessary. (And if you do, don't beat yourself up about it. You may have wanted a water birth surrounded by scented candles and CDs of whale songs, but ended up with an emergency C-section. It's not ideal, but all that really matters is that the baby and Mum are okay.)

Choosing a location
You have three choices:
- *Hospital birth*: This is the most common choice for pregnant women; about 94 per cent of mums have their babies in hospital.
- *Midwife-led birthing unit*: A less clinical setting than a hospital; more of a home from home. Care is provided by midwives. Not all areas of the country offer this option.
- *Home birth*: Around two in a hundred women choose to have their babies at home.

A recent study published in the *British Medical Journal* indicates that for women with low risk pregnancies the overall risk to Mum and baby remains low in all settings. But if you have a complication in your pregnancy or your pregnancy is considered to be a high risk, you may have no choice and have to deliver in hospital.

Where to deliver is a very personal choice. Some women worry about the idea of not having the baby in a hospital; conversely, other women want to avoid the clinical setting and deliver at home.

Tip: Read up on the options and ask your midwife for guidance as well on the services and facilities on offer in your area. Go and have a look around at the hospital and birth centre so that you can make an informed decision. Also speak to other mums, and see how they found their birth location.

Thinking about pain relief
I cover pain relief options in the later section 'Easing the pain'. It's worth taking a look at that section and considering the options for pain relief before you go into labour. And if you want to use a TENS machine, you need to buy or hire one in advance.

Considering types of delivery
There are several ways you can deliver:
- *Active birth*: Most women give birth 'naturally' – they push the baby out, and the midwife catches her.
- *Caesarean*: The baby is removed from the womb during a surgical procedure. The National Institute for Clinical Excellence has recently changed its guidelines to allow pregnant women in the UK an elective caesarean if they still want it following a discussion with mental health experts. Until now, caesareans were only permitted for medical reasons. Note: Make sure you know all the information about the pros and cons of vaginal versus caesarean birth before opting for a caesarean. A caesarean is a major operation, with a long recovery period.
- *Water birth*: At home, or in your local hospital or birth centre, if they have the facility, you can give birth in a water pool. Water eases some of the pain of childbirth (you can also use a water pool for pain relief initially, and then deliver out of the water).

You need to decide on how you want to deliver weeks before the birth, but do remember that if baby or Mum needs it, the best laid plans can change during delivery.

'Dads, advice if you're thinking of getting in the birthing pool with your partner: 1) Check you're allowed first, don't just jump in. 2) Wear baggy shorts, not a Speedo. 3) Beware floaty things.'
Jason, dad to Harry

Deciding on a birth partner

Some hospitals and birthing centres allow only one birth partner; some allow two. Many women have their partners at their side, both for support and to help Dad bond with the baby. Some mums have a mum, sister, friend or doula (a doula is a lady experienced in childbirth whom you hire to support you through birth, and sometimes afterwards as well).

What Mum is looking for in a birth partner is someone who can cope in a crisis, who makes her feel calm, whom she listens to and who she thinks can advocate on her behalf – for example tell a midwife she really doesn't want her to do something if she's struggling to make her feelings known. Often, mums who've already given birth make great support buddies for the delivery.

You may have read the previous paragraph and thought, oh dear, that doesn't sound like the father. Perhaps not, but if Dad wants to be at the birth and Mum wants him there, have faith in Dad. When it's the woman you love giving birth to your child, you find the strength and courage from somewhere.

'To be honest, I was worried about James being at the birth, because he's hopeless with medical stuff. He fainted once just getting his blood pressure taken. But he came with me to all the scans and appointments (he had to leave the room for blood tests), and I knew I wanted him to see the moment his son was born. On the day, he was brilliant. He just focused on me, rather than the medical stuff going on. And it was so great to see him hold Caleb for the first time.'
Gemma, mum to Caleb

Packing your baby bags

It's a good idea to have some bags packed ready for when you go into labour – in case you don't have time to potter about the house packing up on the day. Most women do this around week 36. (Even if you plan to deliver at home, pack a bag just in case.)

Tip: Pack three bags – one for the Mum and Dad during birth, one for Mum after the birth and one for baby after birth. It's not ideal being in labour at the hospital and mid-contraction trying to find the TENS machine at the bottom of a suitcase full of nappies and babygros.

In Mum and Dad's labour bag, you could include books and magazines (to keep you distracted); a camera/camcorder; dressing gown, socks and slippers; items to make Mum feel more at home and/or for Mum to focus on during contractions – for example, a cushion or a photo; maternity pads – plenty of them; music you want to listen to during the birth; a nightdress – one you don't mind getting messy; snacks and drinks; and a TENS machine, if you're using one.

In Mum's after-birth bag, consider including breast pads, clothes to wear home, a comfy bra, ear plugs (hospital wards can be very noisy), lots of maternity pads, phone numbers so you can tell people baby's arrived, plenty of spare underwear (not your best knickers), pyjamas or nighties, and a washbag.

And in your baby's bag, pop in cotton wool, hats, muslin cloths, nappies, scratch mitts, sleepsuits, socks, a teddy or comforter and vests.

Don't fret about having forgotten something; the hospital has supplies and Dad can pop home and get things.

Trying different methods to bring on labour

Your baby is considered full term at 37 weeks, but many doctors prefer that women deliver from 39 weeks onwards, to ensure the baby's lungs are sufficiently mature.

So, from 39 weeks onwards – and especially if you go past your due date and the midwife is talking about induction – many women are keen for the baby to come, and they try different techniques to bring on labour.

Here are some methods you can try:
- Bouncing on a gym/birthing ball.
- Eating curry – supposedly, a spicy curry stimulates your intestines, and, in turn, your uterus.
- Eating fresh pineapple – said to soften the cervix.
- Having sex – not easy to find a position that works by late pregnancy, but sex (and especially an orgasm) can trigger the release of the hormone oxytocin, which starts contractions.
- Stimulating your nipples – rubbing nipples (like a baby feeds) can lead to oxytocin release.
- Taking castor oil – but be careful, it can make you sick.
- Taking raspberry leaf in a tea or tablet.
- Walking or doing housework – pushes the baby down onto the cervix, which can stimulate oxytocin release.

Don't get too het up about making labour start; your baby will come when she's good and ready. But as long as you try them in moderation (don't eat 14 pineapples a day), the methods above can't hurt.

Getting checked out when you have concerns

No one wants to be seen as a hypochondriac, but when you're pregnant with your first child, you don't know what to expect – and you're naturally concerned for the baby.

If you're worried about symptoms you have, or you haven't felt your baby move much recently, you're not wasting anyone's time by asking for a check-up. Hearing your baby's heartbeat on the monitor really puts your mind at ease.

You may also be worried about knowing the difference between early labour contractions and Braxton Hicks contractions – tightening of the muscles in the womb that can happen from time to time from mid-pregnancy. Labour contractions are longer, stronger, more painful and more regular. But if you're having contractions that are painful, best to get checked.

KNOWING WHAT TO EXPECT DURING CHILDBIRTH

Knowledge is power against the fear of the unknown. Your best preparation for childbirth is to learn about what's going to happen.

Going into labour

Being in labour means having contractions that dilate the cervix ready for birth. Early labour may start as cramps or lower backache, or you may feel fine until the first contraction.

Your midwife will have advised you when to call the midwife or labour suite during your labour. If you've had a complication in pregnancy, or your waters have broken, you may need to go straight to hospital. Otherwise, you may be advised to stay at home, where you're more comfortable, and wait until the contractions are really picking up and you're in active labour (see the next section 'Knowing how labour progresses').

> 'Looking back, I realise I was probably in labour for a day or so before I realised it. I'd had such awful backache, but I assumed I'd just overdone it.'
> Katie, mum to Barney

Knowing how labour progresses

Here's an outline of the stages of labour:

1. *Early labour.* Labour begins. Contractions may start off as mild cramps, and then get stronger and closer together. The cervix begins to dilate. Unless you need to go to hospital for a medical reason, you can stay home during this stage and carry on, pretty much as normal.

2. *Active phase.* Labour intensifies. During this phase the cervix opens right up. Contractions are stronger – they build

up to a climax and then dissipate. They can be as frequent as every few minutes and last up to a minute and a half.

3.   *Transitional phase*: You're moving towards the pushing stage now. The cervix fully dilates to ten centimetres (which is how wide it needs to be for baby to come through). Women respond differently in this phase – you may be irritable or sick or shaky.

4.   *Birth*: You have the urge to push and do so with contractions. There are a variety of positions in which you can give birth, but those in which gravity lends a hand are best. With each push your baby moves down a little more. Every birth is different – some babies come out after a few pushes; some take their time.

Through the birth the midwife monitors both Mum and your baby to make sure everything's going okay. If either gets into difficulties, medical intervention may be necessary (see the later section 'Getting a helping hand').

Easing the pain
You may have some pretty firm views on pain relief already. The best advice you'll hear on pain relief is this: be prepared to be flexible.

No woman knows what it feels like to be in labour until she is. You don't know how you'll feel, and how you'll cope with contractions and birth. The kindest thing you can do for yourself is to be open to needing some support during labour. You may start off determined to deliver with just a TENS machine and some gas and air; but don't make it a rigid rule.

Here are the various options of pain relief available to women in labour:

•   *Epidural*: These are only available for hospital births. A small catheter is inserted into the spinal column and a drug is injected in. Depending on the type of epidural, the lower part of your body may be numb, or you may be able to walk about.

- *Gas and air.* You breathe in entonox (a mix of oxygen and nitrous oxide) while having a contraction, and it has a calming effect and takes the edge off the pain.
- *Drugs.* The usual option is pethedine, a painkiller and relaxant. It's delivered by injection.
- *TENS machine.* Delivers small electrical pulses to pads attached to your back. As labour intensifies, you control the strength and frequency of the pulses in line with contractions. Sounds bizarre, but I found it very helpful.

It's beyond the scope of this book to go into detail on how each option works and its possible side effects. Your midwife will be able to guide you on each option.

Also consider natural pain relief options – taking a warm bath, massage, using a birth ball, finding comfortable positions, using breathing exercises, hypnobirthing (self-hypnosis).

> 'TENS machine was brilliant. It really helped my partner in the early stages, and it gave me something to do to help her rather than standing about helplessly.'
> Adam, dad to Claire

Getting a helping hand
Sometimes, with the best will in the world, Mum needs some help giving birth – perhaps because she's too tired to push any more, because the baby's got herself into an awkward position like breech (feet first) or because her heartbeat is dropping and it's essential to get her out fast. Mum may feel pretty upset at the thought of medical intervention, but the midwives and doctors know best, and what counts is getting the baby out safely.

Here are some of the ways in which midwives and doctors sometimes help Mum along:
- *Induction.* If Mum's body is showing no signs of going into labour by a certain point, a midwife may recommend that she be induced. Inductions occur for three reasons: Mum's gone past 41 weeks; labour hasn't started after the waters

break; in cases of a chronic condition, such as pre-eclampsia or diabetes. There are various ways to bring on labour; here they are listed in the order they're carried out (if one doesn't work, you may move on to the next):

• *Membrane sweep*: The midwife does an internal exam during which she tries to separate the membrane surrounding the baby from the cervix, which can bring on labour.

• *Prostaglandin*: Another internal, during which the midwife puts this hormone-like stuff on your cervix.

• *Syntocinon*: A hormone delivered intravenously via a drip.

• *Breaking the waters*: Sometimes, when labour is progressing slowly, the midwife will pierce the membrane around the baby, breaking the waters.

• *Episiotomy*: A surgical cut between the back passage and the vagina. Sorry, but there's no more delicate way to put it! The midwife may suggest this if the baby's getting distressed and needs to come out quickly, or if she thinks you're going to tear badly.

• *Ventouse or forceps*: Called an 'assisted birth', the midwife pulls the baby out, while Mum pushes, with the help of either a ventouse (a little vacuum that attaches to the baby's head) or forceps (a little like salad tongs, but designed to fit around your baby's head).

If your baby is really distressed, you may need to go for an unplanned C-section. This takes place in an operating theatre. Unless the C-section is an emergency and you don't have an epidural in place ready, Mum's usually awake for the procedure and Dad is usually allowed in – so you can both see baby be born.

The moment you've all been waiting for, and beyond
When you ask most women what they remember most about labour, they tell you it's the actual birth – the moment when the baby comes into the world. The emotions you feel when your baby slips out into the midwife or doctor's hands are so strong –

relief, joy, love, pride. That moment makes the labour worthwhile.

Your baby might cry when she emerges; or she may not. George gave a little bark of surprise and then looked about grumpily.

Tip: Something to prepare yourself for: your baby's going to be kind of gross-looking at first. Her skin may be a bit bluish or crimson, her head may be a bit pointy, her nose may be a bit squished, her genitals may be swollen and she'll be covered in all sorts of bodily substances. Don't panic – in a few days, after a good wash and a chance to recover from the birth process, she'll be just beautiful.

The midwife can put the baby straight on Mum's chest if she wants – research has shown that skin-to-skin contact right after birth has all sorts of benefits, from helping parent and child to bond to stabilising the baby's temperature, breathing and heart rate. During that time you may be asked whether you want to cut the umbilical cord – a job for Dad perhaps. Within the first few minutes the midwife or doctor will check the baby twice against the criteria of the Apgar scale (skin colour, heart rate, reflex response, muscle tone and breathing) to see how she's doing. Then she'll take her aside for a minute or two to check her over, clean her up a bit and weigh her.

'How I first felt when I held Emile: overjoyed, yet overawed at the responsibility ahead of me. Exhilarated, yet terrified. Complete, in an inexplicable spiritual sense. Extremely giddy with happiness.'
John, dad to Emile and Gabriel

' "Well, that nose doesn't come from my side of the family" is what I said after Ava was born; she was a bit battered after a ventouse delivery and had a nose like a boxer, but of course it corrected itself in time!'
Sam, dad to Ava

Now, in an ideal world that would be where this section ended: happy Mum and Dad, beautiful new baby. However, there's still a little way to go before Mum's all sorted.

First, Mum needs to deliver the placenta. Most hospitals offer mums an injection which speeds the final stage of the birth process, and allows the placenta to come out without Mum needing to push. Once the placenta's out, the midwife makes sure she's got it all and checks that there's no more bleeding than there should be.

Then, if Mum has torn or had an episiotomy during the labour, the midwife examines the cut and sees whether Mum needs stitches. Even as I write the words, I'm cringing, because I can imagine how an expectant mum reading this feels. Really, don't worry! First of all, tearing is very common (according to the Royal College of Obstetricians and Gynaecologists, up to 90 per cent of women tear to some extent during childbirth), and to be honest it's all lost amid the other discomfort and the sensations of childbirth. And I found, with a local anesthetic and a nice dose of gas and air, I didn't feel the midwife stitching at all; and anyway, I was too busy gazing at my baby boy thinking victoriously, *I did it*!

Finally, when Mum's good to go, and if she can manage, then it's time for a trip to the shower to clean up; and then back to bed for a rest, some tea and toast, some quality family time and your baby's first feed (for more on the first feed, head to Chapter 5).

SOME ADVICE FOR DADS
Although I've written this chapter for both mums and dads, dads commonly feel a bit lost on the sidelines during labour and birth – 'this woman's work'. And the whole experience can lead to emotional overload.

I went into labour in the evening, right before *Match of the Day*, not an ideal start for my husband. A couple of hours later he was ushered out of the labour ward and told to go home and get some rest – because it was my first baby, it was bound to be a slow one. At 5.30 a.m., he was phoned and told to come right away as I was pushing. He hurtled up to the hospital and rushed into the delivery room, only to be confronted by the sight of his wife huffing and puffing and saying most unladylike things at an impressive volume. It was quite a shock. He had a little lie down on the delivery room floor for a couple of minutes, and then felt much better and was up and chanting 'Push' with the midwives.

Here are some tips for Dad to help you get through what's no doubt the most worrying experience of your life:

•   Don't worry if your beautiful, lovely, loving partner morphs into some terrifying monster from a horror film during birth. She'll soon be back to normal. And, in time, you'll regain use of the hand she's crushed mid-contraction.

•   If feeling helpless, do something practical– massage her back, wipe her face with a cool flannel, plump her pillows.

•   Keep encouraging your partner through the whole process; she's more likely to listen to you than anyone.

•   Tell her she's beautiful, tell her she's amazing, tell her she's ever so brave, tell her she's the strongest person you know – tell her anything that lets her know you love her and that she can do this.

•   Once the baby's born, it can be overwhelming, and the first time you hold your baby you may be scared that you'll drop her or get it wrong. Women tend to have more experience with babies than men, so it's understandable it you feel reticent. My husband spent the first day carrying George around on a pillow like he was Cinderella's slipper. Do whatever feels comfortable, and trust that you have the natural instincts you need as a father.

'It was an amazing experience. I don't know whether I was much help. I think I irritated her quite a lot, judging by her snapping. But I was so glad I was there for her, and to see Holly born. I look at Anna in a whole new light now. Women are heroes!'
Steve, dad to Holly

'Steve's right, he was annoying. He kept counting down when I was having a contraction, and he was obsessed with me sucking ice cubes. I hate ice cubes. But I was glad he was there. Now when he has man flu I say to him, "One word for you: childbirth." And he gets it.'
Anna, mum to Holly

COPING WHEN THINGS DIDN'T GO TO PLAN

Hopefully, you find birth a positive experience, and once you hold your baby in your arms the experience of labour fades into the background.

But you may find you have negative feelings about the birth – you feel angry or upset or traumatised by the experience, perhaps because it didn't go as you wanted (you had an assisted birth or an emergency caesarean, for example) or because it was a frightening and painful time.

It's important to understand that this is normal; you're not weak or a coward for reacting this way. Labour is so-named for a reason – it's hard, draining work.

The best thing you can do is to share how you feel with people – your partner, your family, your friends, your midwife/health visitor. Talking about emotions helps, as does others' comfort and reassurance. But if you find you're unable to talk to others, or that your feelings are overwhelming, take a look at the section on birth trauma in Chapter 14.

Finally, try to focus on the outcome of the experience rather than the experience itself. A moment stroking your baby's soft, downy head and gazing at her tiny, perfect features can be very healing.

IF ONLY SOMEONE HAD TOLD ME: ADVICE FROM PARENTS

- Don't bother fretting about your bikini line before birth; once you're in labour, you'll lose all embarrassment over people looking at your lady bits. Leave your dignity in a carrier bag by the door on the way into the hospital and collect it again on the way out.

• Doing a little physical work (walking, hoovering and so on) to try to bring on labour is one thing; doing a marathon cleaning session is another. Bear in mind that you don't want to wear yourself out before labour even begins.

• Dad, give the gas and air a miss. You may find the nitrous oxide (laughing gas) hilarious; Mum likely won't. And you don't want to annoy a woman in labour.

• Sometimes, while pushing, a little something else slips out from a different passage, if you get the drift. Don't worry; midwifes have seen it all.

• Remember to breathe while pushing. If you hold your breath – as you may instinctively do – there's less oomph in your push.

• You know the saying 'What happens on tour, stays on tour'? Well, the same goes for childbirth. Whatever happens in the delivery room, stays in the delivery room – unless both parents are happy to share.

4. Settling into life as a parent

This chapter focuses on the first six weeks or so of baby's life. This is a period during which you do most of your adjusting and learning as a parent – where you start to get the hang of this parenting malarkey. They're precious weeks, as you spend lots of time getting to know your baby, and he builds a relationship with you. Also be sure to check out Chapter 5 as well, which covers milk feeding – a key concern for new parents in the first weeks.

ADJUSTING IN THE FIRST FEW DAYS
Holy moly – you're a parent! It's a big deal, and you're likely to feel a bit in shock for the first few days (especially given that you've just been through a dramatic event – the birth).
    Here are some things it's normal to think/feel:
- Hooray, pregnancy is over!
- Hooray, the birth is behind us!
- I feel suffocated by the baby's neediness.
- I love my baby so much.
- I miss my life before baby.
- I miss time with my partner.
- It gets easier. Tell me it gets easier.
- My partner's so focused on the baby now; what about me?
- Oh wow, I can't believe I have a baby.
- Sleeping, feeding, pooping, crying – is this all he does?
- Tiny toes, tiny fingers, perfect.
- Why did I want a baby! This is exhausting!
- Why don't they come with a mute/off switch?
- Will I ever sleep again?

As you can see, you'll probably think/feel a mix of things, both positive and negative. And that's fine. It doesn't mean you don't love your baby. It doesn't mean you aren't now or won't be in the future a good parent.

Myth buster. All parents feel instant delight and adoration at becoming a parent, right? Well no, not all parents feel connected to the baby at once. Sometimes, bonding takes a little time. Just as you may not fall in love at first sight with a partner, sometimes parents need some time to get to know their babies before they feel really connected. That's okay. You get there in the end.

RECOVERING FROM THE BIRTH

It's sad that our culture has evolved not to provide much help to a new mother. In many cultures around the world a new mother is revered and pampered, and so it used to be in the UK, with mothers encouraged to stay in hospital for a week after birth and take some time to recover while having help with the baby. Nowadays, Mum may be heading home within hours of the baby's birth, and while you may have an army of relatives on hand to help you and a mum or mother-in-law prepared to move in for some weeks, many couples go home to an empty house.

Such was the case for my husband and me, and I remember thinking that with what my body had been through, it was nuts to be home and trying to care for a tiny baby. But if you don't have the choice to sit back and be mothered yourself, you need to find a way to get through as your body and mind recover from the birth experience – lots of rest, let Dad help out (and dads, please do help out!), be as kind to yourself as you can.

Physically, you may feel pretty sore. It gets better – honest! (Otherwise no woman would ever have sex again!) Take each day as it comes, take what painkillers you're allowed and get as much rest as you can.

Tip: Many women swear by arnica tablets (available from large pharmacies) to help the body heal after birth.

Also be prepared for some see-sawing emotions. 'Baby blues' are common in the first few days, and are caused by your hormones shifting about.

'I took a lot of baths after the birth. The bleeding after-wards used to make me feel icky, and baths helped me feel fresh – plus it was a little me time, and it relaxed me. David used to have Henry, or I'd just pop him in his bouncy chair by the bath. As he got older, I started taking him in with me, and he loved it.'
Karen, mum to Henry

A NOTE ON SLEEP
Chapter 8 is entirely devoted to sleep – because it's a big deal in the first year. But it's worth touching on sleep here too, because what stands out for most parents in the first few weeks is the lack of sleep.

Newborns haven't a clue when they're meant to be sleeping, and because their tummies are so tiny, they needed to be filled regularly – and I'm afraid this means during the night.

Some newborns sleep for four or five hours in one go during the night; some are up every couple of hours. Regardless of your baby's sleeping, you're going to get tired – especially Mum, whose body is recovering from a major physical event. Which is why you need to take it easy in these first weeks. Leave the gallivant-ing until the baby's a bit older, and sleep when you can in the day.

And if you're feeling down, remember that sleep deprivation is playing a big part in this. And it will get better. One day you'll have a child who goes to bed early evening and sleeps until morning. And you'll appreciate the night's sleep you get all the more!

'When Edward was a week old, my mother came to visit. Edward was so unsettled – you'd get him to sleep then he'd wake up again soon after. She thought it might be that he was waking himself up moving in his sleep, and freaking out at the feel of the space around him. She showed me how to swaddle him in a thin baby blanket, so his arms and legs were tucked in tight like in the womb.

He slept so much better after that. He was like a bug in a rug.'
Kate, mum to Edward

(See Chapter 8 for instructions on how to swaddle your baby.)

REALISING THAT IT GETS EASIER

The first few weeks are the toughest – it's going to get easier from here. I remember my godmother saying to me when George was a couple of weeks old that there are milestones at which you realise it's getting easier – six weeks, three months, six months, one year, and I agree.

In the first six weeks your baby is at his most unsettled and needy, and both Mum and Dad are tired and dealing with the huge practical and emotional adjustment of becoming a parent. In a few weeks the baby and his parents have got to know each other, and established some form of normality in their new life together. You go from fumbling over sleepsuit poppers to effortlessly snapping your baby into his pjs; from wrestling with the car seat to knowing just how to slot it in; from struggling to get your baby's wind up to knowing just what works to get an almighty, satisfying burp – you go from feeling out of your depth to feeling a building confidence that you know how to look after your baby.

And if these first few weeks are a struggle for you, focus on that six-week marker. Because along with it comes your baby's first smile – and that makes all the tiredness and the worry and the confusion pale into the background.

Tip for mums: As time goes on, if you really don't feel that you're coping, or you feel down or are struggling with your feelings towards your baby, take a look at Chapter 14, where I discuss the signs of post-natal depression.

'Babies go through lots of phases, some good and some not so enjoyable, but they don't usually last. My baby seemed to be a very cross little person during the first eight weeks of her life. This was partly due, I think, to hunger. I was desperately trying to get the hang of breast-feeding but it just wasn't meant to be. Once we resolved this and I stopped feeling guilty about it she was much happier and so was I. Other examples are where you might think you baby will never sleep through but they all do. There are also colic, clingy phases and "I don't want a bath!" phases. These things tend to come and go. Be patient.'

Sarah, mum to Scarlet

GETTING TO GRIPS WITH THE BASICS OF BABY CARE

Having touched on the emotional impact of baby's arrival, now let's take a look at some of the practicalities of caring for baby. Often, this is the kind of stuff parents beat themselves up for not knowing or handling expertly at first – but unless you have experience with babies, why would you a clue what to do with one! A lot of bringing up a baby is innate, instinctive in you; knowing how to cut his nails or put on a nappy isn't.

Bathing

The recommendation is to use only water on a newborn baby's skin, because it's so sensitive. You can use cotton wool soaked in water to wash your baby, and you can bath him in a baby bath, basin, sink or your own big bath. Your baby may not be impressed the first time he takes a bath, but he soon gets used to it – remember, he's used to the sensation of being surrounded by fluid from his time in the womb, and a bath can be comforting. Make sure the water's not too hot – use your elbow to test it – and don't keep him in for long or he gets cold.

Tip: One of the easiest ways to bath baby is to put a bath mat or towel at the bottom of the bath, run a little water and lie baby on the mat/towel on his back. Then you have both hands free to swoosh water over him.

Clothing

Newborn babies don't regulate their temperature as well as we do, so it's important to keep your baby warm. But that doesn't mean you dress your baby in loads of layers to the point that he overheats (which is dangerous for baby). Feel your baby's skin (on the back of the neck is best) to gauge whether he's hot, cold or just right.

> 'I had so many outfits for Chloe. But in the end when she was little I found it easier to just dress her in sleepsuits – they kept her warm, they had built in scratch mitts and they were easy to get on and off once I got the hang of it.'
> Jess, mum to Chloe

Crying

All babies cry. It's their only means of communication. If your baby cries it usually means one of these things: he's hungry, he's wet/dirty, he's cold/hot, he's ill/in pain, he's tired, he's over-stimulated, he fancies a cuddle. You soon get to hear the difference in your baby's cry – for example, a hungry George cry sounded ferocious and furious; a 'Mum, can I have a snuggle' cry sounded more whimper-like.

Some babies develop colic, which is typically characterised by long bouts of crying that you just can't soothe, usually at the same time of day (often evenings), sometimes combined with pulling his legs up to his tummy. Experts don't quite agree on the cause of colic – some think it's tummy ache because baby's system is struggling to cope with digestion; some think it's down to wind; some believe the crying is due to the baby's immature nervous system – that he's simply overloaded. Colic can start from two to three weeks, and usually lasts a few weeks at most.

Tip: It's miserable having a baby with colic. If your baby's crying is getting too much for you, put him down in a safe place (for example his crib or basket) and take five minutes to yourself. Of course you want to be there for your baby, but if you're not coping, you're not helping your baby by sticking it out. He'll be fine for a few minutes while you make a cup of tea or just sit somewhere else in the house and calm down.

Tip: If your baby has colic, try wearing ear plugs while you sit with him. It's the volume and the intensity of the cry that is most hard to bear, and diffusing the noise helps you cope.

Some babies cry and cry and cry. The organisation Cry-sis (www.cry-sis.org.uk) offers support if you're struggling to cope with your baby's crying.

Holding your baby
Babies seem so fragile, and at first you may feel quite anxious when holding your baby. You'll soon gain confidence.

There are two areas of the baby you must really pay attention to:

• *Neck*: A tiny baby can't support the weight of his head. Left unsupported, his neck won't hold up the head, and his head can loll about. Always prop up his neck when he's little.
• *Head*: Babies have two soft spots on their head called fontanelles. The one on the top of the head is large and quite easy to feel and closes over between twelve and eighteen months after birth; the one on the back is smaller and closes quickly (in six weeks after birth). These soft spots are Nature's clever trick to help the baby's large head fit through the birth canal – the connective tissue squishes up during the birth, allowing the bones around the fontanelles to move closer, meaning the baby's head changes shape and is smaller in circumference. Of course you're going to protect your baby's head in any case and make sure he doesn't bump it, but it's worth remembering that these spots are fragile areas where your baby doesn't yet have bone protecting his brain.

There are all sorts of way to hold a young baby – upright with his tummy to your chest and his head up by your shoulder, so he can look behind you; cradled in your arms horizontally; in a seated position with his back to your chest – one hand under his bottom as a seat, the other across his chest to keep him secure (but not sitting on your hip – only older babies who can hold up their heads reliably can manage this). Relax, and in time you'll find what feels comfortable for you and your little one (he'll soon tell you if he doesn't like a position!).

Nappies

Whether you're using disposables or reusables, you may at first struggle to do up a nappy, but you soon get the hang of it. Do it up too loose and your baby wriggles out; do it up too tight and your baby's uncomfortable; leave the leg bits skew-whiff and your baby leaks. And as you wipe your baby, remember to wipe the back end and front end separately to avoid cross-infection.

So how often do you change baby? Well, a newborn may wee or poo quite regularly, so the usual advice is to change baby after a feed, and when he does a poo.

Tip: If baby keeps nodding off during his feed, and you want him to take more so he'll go longer before his next feed, change his nappy mid-feed. It wakes him up, and then he'll take some more milk.

Nails

Newborns often have sharp nails, and that's why scratch mitts were invented – to stop your baby scratching himself while flailing his arms around. You don't need to cut your baby's nails until he's six to eight weeks old (cut them too early and you may make him bleed and cause infection). When you do come to cut them, teeny baby nail clippers work well.

ACCEPTING HELP

Newborns are hard work, and add to that Mum recovering from birth and both Mum and Dad wondering where their time for each other has gone and you have a recipe for meltdown.

There are lots of ways you can let people help in these early weeks – from doing household chores like cooking, shopping and cleaning to watching the baby while you have a rest or some time to yourself or with your partner.

A NOTE ON VISITORS

It's part of our culture to visit a new baby and welcome it to the world. So you can expect plenty of people to want to come and see your new baby.

Remember that it's your right to choose who comes, and if you're feeling overwhelmed, either ask someone to come once the baby's older, or if they're already visiting, to suggest it's time to go. Your visitors should respect that as a parent you need a little space with your baby at the start.

Also watch how much your baby is passed about people. If he's happy with it, great. But if he's starting to show signs of being tired, or over-stimulated, suggest it's time he took a nap. Mums in particular may also find it hard to see other people hold the baby because there's such a strong natural instinct to keep him close. Hopefully, your visitors have the sensitivity to pick up on Mum getting antsy and hand the baby back; if not, ask nicely but firmly.

Finally, make sure your baby doesn't come into contact with poorly people, because his immune system isn't ready to take on bugs – so if friends or family members want to visit but have a cold or cough or tummy upset, ask them to reschedule.

CHECK-UPS FOR MUM AND THE BABY

Your baby goes through a number of routine health checks in the first six weeks – some right after birth, some a few days later, some at a six-week check. Here are the areas the midwife and doctor look at:

- *Physical examination* – top-to-toe after birth, and focusing in on eyes, heart, hips and testicles in boys. Also looks out for jaundice (shows as a yellowish tinge to the skin) which is common in newborns.

- *Hearing test.*
- *Blood test* (taken from the baby's heel), to check for various conditions including sickle cell disease and cystic fibrosis.

Care differs between local authorities, but in most you can expect the following:

- *Midwife visit:* You might have a midwife visit in the first couple of days that you're home with your baby, to see how you're coping and to check how the baby's doing.
- *Health visitor.* The midwife hands you over to a health visitor, whose job is to give advice on caring for your baby. She gives you a red book for the baby in which all health information is recorded.
- *GP check-up:* At around six weeks, Mum and the baby go to see the doctor for a post-natal check-up. As well as checking the baby's vitals, the doctor takes Mum's blood pressure, feels Mum's stomach to check the womb has contracted as it should and, if she had a caesarean, checks the wound. Depending on circumstances, Mum may also have further tests, such as a blood test. If you have any concerns about how your body is post-birth, this is the time to share them.

As well as these routine check-ups, you'll be invited to attend regular weighing sessions to check how the baby's developing – often at first, and then with decreasing frequency as your baby gets older. At the sessions health visitors are usually on hand to answer any questions you may have. You weigh your baby, and chart his weight in the red book on a graph that shows you how he's doing. The point of the weighing session is to check that the baby is thriving and gaining weight well. If your baby's weight gain is outside of the healthy range then your health visitor can discuss feeding with you and see how to help your baby gain the weight he needs.

'My tips for the first weeks:
1.   Get as much sleep as you can.

2.   Make life easier for yourself – use baby wipes for cleaning!

3.   Ask for help – everyone wants to help in these early weeks.

4.   Don't say you will never do anything, for example a dummy. You may regret it later when the baby is screaming at 4 a.m. and you haven't had a good night's sleep for days.

5.   Lower your expectations.

6.   Don't try to be a super person. Sod the washing up, leaving it's not going to kill you.'

Emma, mum to Joshua

IF ONLY SOMEONE HAD TOLD ME: ADVICE FROM PARENTS

•   Everyone says it, and it's good advice: sleep when the baby sleeps.

•   Pulling a soiled baby vest over the baby's head isn't the way to go.

•   Baby boys have an impressive range when weeing, and will do so at the most inopportune times.

•   If the baby's in a right old mess with a dirty nappy, hose him down in the sink.

•   Forget fancy skincare products. Open your kitchen cupboard, grab the olive oil, and rub a little into baby's skin if he has a dry patch.

•   Always have spare baby clothes! Exploding poos (pootastrophes) can happen anywhere.

•   Some babies get spots after birth. Resist the urge to squeeze!

•   If you can't get your baby to settle, try a drive in the car or a ride on top of the washing machine. Rhythmic vibrations often help.

•   Everyone has an opinion on what you should do with your baby. Use what you like ('Here's a great way to burp') and discard what you don't ('That baby is tired. I can tell. Hadn't you better put that baby in his cot?').

5. Milk feeds and your baby

You feed a baby purely on milk from birth until around six months of age (you can wean from 16 weeks), and then slowly decrease milk feeds as you increase solid food, until at the age of one the baby is eating three meals a day and snacks and perhaps just having milk a couple of times a day, such as first thing and bedtime. (To find out about food and weaning, head to Chapter 7.) That's a lot of milk that a baby drinks in year one! This chapter gives you the lowdown on milk feeding, covering how you feel about feeding, how you feed your baby (bottle or breast) and when (feed-on-demand or routine).

RELAXING ABOUT FEEDING

Before getting into the nitty gritty of feeding, it's worth thinking about your overall approach.

Parents can get pretty stressed about feeding – is your baby drinking enough milk? Too much? The best thing you can do when it comes to your baby's feeding is chill out. The tenser you are, the harder it is for your baby to relax. Yes, if you're concerned about your baby's feeding have a chat with a health visitor or doctor; but don't blow it out of proportion and get fixated on every drop that passes your baby's lips.

When it comes to feeding, your baby knows best. If your baby's full, she stops feeding. If she's hungry, she soon lets you know. It's not always easy to let your baby lead the way with feeding, especially if you think she should be feeding more or less. But working with your baby, rather than pushing her, makes for a happier relationship between you and your baby, and between baby and food.

Of course, this advice applies to babies who are normal feeders/eaters – by which I mean there's no real cause for concern. If your baby isn't thriving or gaining weight, has a reflux problem or simply refuses to wean, for example, you need to be guided by your doctor's advice.

Flexibility is also key – be prepared to adapt the approach you've decided to adopt for feeding if it doesn't suit your baby or you, or even to ditch it entirely. For example, you may be determined to breastfeed, but encounter difficulties and move to part breastfeeding and part bottle-feeding.

As with all aspects of parenting, you need to let go of judgement and guilt, and be willing to experiment. It really doesn't matter what path you choose, as long as it's the one that best fits you and your baby.

GETTING TO GRIPS WITH THE BASICS OF FEEDING

Here's how it works. Your newborn baby will get hungry. You'll realise that she's hungry because she's fretful, and she might also be smacking her lips and rooting about desperately sucking at anything, like your finger (if she's moved on to crying, she's really hungry). You feed your baby, either on the breast or by bottle (see the later sections for details). At first, your baby may take a very long time to feed, as she sucks so slowly. Once she's finished feeding, she'll either look about a bit, or nod off. A couple of hours later, you'll start the process again.

As your baby gets older, she'll take more milk, drink it in a shorter space of time, and will be able to go longer between feeds.

Sounds simple, and it would be but for the issue of wind. Little babies swallow lots of air as they feed (especially bottle-fed babies), and that air needs to come back out or they get that horrid 'Help, I'm going to pop' feeling (you know, the one you get when you drink too much fizzy soda in one go). If you don't burp your baby during and after a feed, she's likely to feed less (because she feels full), she can be in pain when you lay her down (so refuse to sleep) and when she does burp you may well get a faceful of milky reflux.

There are all kinds of ways to burp a baby – the golden rule for all is to make sure you support the baby's neck:

• Sit her on your knee and hold her up by placing the crook between your index finger and thumb under her jaw – so you're supporting her head from the front (don't throttle her; allow her chin to sit on your hand). Then you have the other hand free to gently pat her back.

• Put your hands around the top of her torso, pushing your fingers up behind her neck so you support the neck. Then gently, and in small movements, twist her torso from side to side.

• Hold her upright, tummy against your chest, so that her head is on your shoulder. Support her bottom with one hand, and with the other rub her back in a circular motion.

A note on reflux: some babies are sick. A lot. They're not vomiting and feeling ill with it as an adult would; they just have an immature digestive system which means sometimes milk comes back up. If you're worried about the level of baby's reflux, see the doctor. The best approach to handling those sicky burps? Keep lots of mussies (muslin squares) handy.

GIVING YOUR BABY HER FIRST FEEDS

The following section helps you decide between breast- and bottlefeeding. But this section comes first, because even if you want to bottlefeed, it's worth considering breastfeeding for the first couple of days. Right after giving birth, Mum's breasts produce colostrum, which is the ideal first milk for the baby because it's full of calories and antibodies that help the baby build her immune system. After two to three days Mum's breasts swell up with breast milk, which replaces the colostrum. So even if you don't want to breastfeed after day two or three, doing so at the start has great health benefits for the baby. You can express colostrum for the baby if you prefer not to breastfeed.

MILK FEEDING: BREAST OR BOTTLE?

Your choice for your baby's milk feeds is between breastfeeding and formula milk. Most parents decide which they want to do before birth, but plans can change.

There's a lot of emotion tied up with milk feeding. A mother breastfeeding is the most natural thing in the world, and it's an intimate experience with the child that many women treasure. Unfortunately, while people don't judge a mother for breastfeeding (though they may scowl if she does so in their eyeshot), many people judge a mother who chooses to bottle-feed.

You have the right to make your own decision. You have your reasons one way or the other, and you don't need to justify them to anyone. So if you encounter a bossy 'breastfeeding expert' in the maternity ward who's scolding you for not breastfeeding, don't let her get you down. And Dad, it's Mum's choice. If she really doesn't want to, you need to respect that. If she tries to breastfeed and it doesn't work out, accept that and appreciate that she tried.

I wanted to breastfeed. But when George came, it just didn't work out for us. After a few days I stopped, and I moved on to bottle-feeding. And then I beat myself up for my choice for a good while. Ultimately, I realised my guilt was getting me nowhere. Being a good mum isn't about breastfeeding rather than bottle-feeding – it's about giving the child love and attention and affection and acceptance. The only thing damaging about the bottle-feeding was my getting down about it, which then affected George!

So whatever choice you make, make it with confidence, and then move on with your life.

'I was quite judgemental before I had my baby about women who don't breastfeed. I thought they were selfish and lazy. I was determined to breastfeed. Actually, it hadn't even occurred to me I'd find it hard. But I did. Whatever position I tried, it was sore. And it got to the point I hated it and would dread each feed. So in the end I

moved on to bottles, and it was a total relief, and I was a much happier mum from that day on. Thinking about it, it taught me a bit of a lesson in judging people!'
Sonia, mum to Michael

'I wanted to breastfeed; it just felt right to me. It was fine until Alana was about six months old, and then some of my friends and family started asking me when I was going to stop. They seemed to think it was time to stop, but I didn't want to yet. I ignored them, and I expressed milk when I went back to work so the childminder could feed her, then she had her morning and evening feed. She was 11 months when she stopped – I think because she didn't need it any more because she was eating so much. I was sad that part of being a mummy was over now, but I was happy Alana had made the choice, not me.'
Lexie, mum to Alana

BREASTFEEDING
Nutritious, warm milk on tap: wonderful for the baby, and convenient for you because your baby's milk is ready for her wherever you are, at whatever time of day.

Knowing how to breastfeed
Successful breastfeeding is about both Mum and the baby feeling comfortable. Your baby needs to 'latch on' correctly, which means she draws a big mouthful of breast deep into her mouth. Then, as her jaw moves up and down as she sucks, she stimulates the milk ducts to give milk. To get your baby latched on, she needs her mouth open wide, and her tongue, bottom lip and chin need to touch your breast first. Try to aim her bottom lip as far as you can from the bottom of your nipple.

Some babies latch on easily, Mum's comfy and away you go. But a lot of mums and babies need a helping hand – and usually some practical support is best. If you intend to breastfeed, it's a good idea to stay in hospital overnight so you have midwives on hand to help you.

There are various positions you can use to breastfeed a baby:

- Lying the baby across your lap, propped up on a cushion – either holding her with the opposite arm to the breast she's feeding from or the same arm.
- Holding your baby under your arm, so her head is at your breast and his legs are at your back.
- Lying down, face to face.

Of course you have two breasts, so which do you use when? The easiest approach is to let your baby feed full from one breast. The first milk your baby gets from the breast is foremilk, and it's rather watery. The good stuff (the hindmilk) comes further into the feed, so the longer the baby feeds on one breast, the more hindmilk she gets. If she's still hungry and you've run out of milk on the first breast then you can move the baby to the other breast. When you do your next feed, use the breast the baby didn't feed on fully in the previous feed.

Tip: Between feeds your breasts often leak milk, so have a stack of breast pads handy.

'Equipment for breastfeeding: feeding bras, cushions, breast pads (disposable or cloth reusable), nipple cream. But the most important bit of your breastfeeding kit is a drink for you! Especially in those first few weeks I would find that almost as soon as Rosie latched on it was like all moisture in my body was suddenly drained away – a most peculiar feeling. So because at first I needed both hands and arms to hold Rosie, the best piece of equipment I had was a straw so I could just lean over and drink while she was feeding!'

Angela, mum to Rosie

Expressing and combining milk

You may try expressing milk so someone else can feed your baby; for example, your partner. Breast pumps have advanced in the past few years, and if you're prepared to invest a little, you can ease the experience. In some local authorities you can also borrow or lease breast pumps from the hospital, so it's worth asking your midwife or health visitor.

Mixing breast- and bottle-feeding (whether it's expressed milk in the bottle or formula) is something many women do as the baby gets older. For example, you may breastfeed your baby in the morning and at night, but while she's at nursery she has formula or expressed milk. Combining breast and bottle isn't recommended for newborns because the baby gets confused between the nipple and the teat.

Dealing with discomfort

Hopefully, breastfeeding is a lovely experience and a precious time with your baby. Sometimes it can become sore for Mum for all kinds of reasons (the baby's not latched on well; you have an infection called mastitis; you have more milk than the baby needs and your breasts are engorged; your nipples are sensitive, or hurt because the baby's biting). Many women swear by cooling gel pads that you refrigerate and then put in your bra, or if you're going old school, try cabbage leaves. If you're worried about how your breasts feel, or breastfeeding is painful, talk to your midwife, health visitor or GP.

Breastfeeding in front of people

One of the aspects of breastfeeding that most concerns mums is privacy – feeding in front of other people. By law, mothers in the UK have the right to breastfeed in a public place. A well-placed muslin cloth or shawl or simply perfecting where your top goes lets your baby feed away happily without everyone seeing.

'When Harry was first born, I found it a bit uncomfortable when my wife breastfed. Don't get me wrong; I was happy

that she was. But I wasn't quite sure where to look. Her breasts had always meant something different to me than feeding a baby. So it was a bit of an adjustment. I soon got used to it though, and it felt normal, nice, not weird.'
Jason, dad to Harry

Getting support

Midwives can help you and your baby get the knack of breast-feeding, and health visitors provide ongoing support. Don't be afraid to ask for more support if your current health professional isn't doing enough. You don't want a matron plonking the baby on your bosom and then sailing off, leaving you stuck next time the baby slips off and needs to be latched on. You need to learn for yourself how to help your baby feed in a way that's comfortable for you both.

There are specific organisations set up to help breastfeeding mothers. Take a look at the Useful Resources section at the end of the book for details.

BOTTLE-FEEDING

My favourite thing about bottle-feeding? It allowed my husband to feed George as well. Which meant nice bonding time for them, and a break for me. My least favourite thing about bottle-feeding? The palaver of sterilising and making up bottles!

'I love feeding Matthew. It's like the world goes away and it's just him and me for a while.'
David, dad to Matthew

Knowing how to bottlefeed

It's fairly straightforward: you find a comfortable position cradling your baby in the crook of your arm so that her head is higher than her body (for obvious reasons – would you like to drink lying flat?), and you pop the teat (the rubber spout) of the bottle into her mouth. Off she goes.

Bottlefed babies often gulp in lots of air with the milk. To minimise trapped wind, make sure you keep the bottle inclined at such an angle that the teat is full of milk.

Baby bottles come with different levels of teat. The starter ones have one small hole so that the baby doesn't get a flood of milk in her mouth. As your baby progresses, you move up the teats to those with more holes, and larger ones, so that she can get more milk from the bottle, and faster. How do you tell when it's time to move up a teat? When your baby is taking ages to feed and is sucking and sucking and sucking at the teat to get the milk.

'Both Toby and Alex were very different feeders even though they were both bottle-fed babies. Here are a few tips I would give:

• Don't go out and buy a bumper pack of bottles with matching brand steriliser (which typically only fit their own-brand bottles), as with both Toby and Alex I had to try a few different types of bottle till I found one that they fed from best.

• When either of the boys were poorly and not taking much milk or having un-scheduled feeds I would buy a large carton of made-up formula so that I could just put a couple of ounces in a bottle at a time rather than making up bottles and having to waste milk.

• When you're out and about or on holiday take cold water sterilising tablets with you. They do the job and items are sterile in 15 minutes.

• Both boys suffered with constipation when they were newborn and it's a horribly tense time when all you want is for your baby to do a poo and you so desperately want do whatever you can to help them out. But I would say don't change milk at once; just try to ride through it as with time their tummies get used to the formula.'

Emma, mum to Toby and Alex

Making up formula

When my mother had children, she was free to make up bottles up to a day in advance, pop them in the fridge, and then heat them up when she needed one. These days the government guidelines say that each bottle should be made up individually – a process that takes around 20 minutes if you follow the instructions on the formula box. The thing is, you haven't always got that long to make a bottle, especially during the night (and especially if you follow the advice of one ridiculous health visitor I met who told me to sterilise bottles individually right before a feed as well – add on another 15 minutes then). So bottle-feeding can present quite a problem.

Every mother I know who bottle-fed had her own approach, and you have to find yours. What's important is to use sterilised bottles, make the formula up with hot water to kill any bugs in the powder and not leave the milk lying about for ages before feeding your baby. The rest you decide yourself:

- *Temperature*: Some mums prefer to use warm milk, so it's closer to breast milk; some babies are quite happy with room temperature.
- *Type of bottle*: There are all kinds of baby bottles and teats on the market. I worked my way through a few before finding a kind that seemed to suit George. Cheap bottles are a false economy in my experience; but some of the most expensive ones are over-designed. A mid-range bottle does fine.
- *Type of milk*: Take your midwife or health visitor's advice, but if your baby is unsettled on that first milk, try another.

'My tip for bottle-feeding is to buy a bottle thermos. Then you can keep a feed cool or warm, depending on which way you're doing it. I used to put boiling water in a sterilised bottle and put it in the thermos. Then, an hour or two later when I was out shopping, I would add the formula and then cool it down.'
Shelly, mum to Daniel

CONSIDERING FEED-ON-DEMAND AND ROUTINES

Do you feed your baby whenever she's hungry, or establish a routine? It's really up to you and down to your parenting style (see Chapter 1).

Feed-on-demand means giving your baby a milk feed whenever she's hungry. As your baby gets older, you learn to recognise her cries and know when to offer a feed. Often breastfeeding mums choose to feed on demand, because breastfed babies tend to feed more regularly, and a routine is hard to establish in the early weeks.

At the other end of the spectrum is a feeding routine. Many childcare books lay down routines for feeding, which are intended to help the parent get some normality and structure back into the day. With a routine you determine set feed times for your baby; for example 7 a.m., 10.30 a.m., 2 p.m., 5 p.m., 7 p.m., 10 p.m. and one night feed.

It can really help you to cope with your new baby if you have some kind of routine. But the problem is, your baby doesn't have a clue what you're doing, and it's easy for her to decide, for example, at 1 p.m. that she's starving and demand a feed, and then she's knocked her routine off kilter for the rest of the day. Some parents calmly move on and get the baby back on track; some parents fall apart trying to force the baby to work to a timetable when the baby has other ideas.

Most parents try both approaches, and settle for something in between. For example, I started off feeding on demand and struggled with the chaos, then I moved to a routine and struggled with George's total refusal to slot into it, then I found a compromise, by which I mean I had a rough routine, but it was flexible and I pretty much went with the flow.

Myth buster. You can't put a newborn baby into a routine. She doesn't know night from day, black from white, the postman from the dog, let alone when she's 'meant' to be hungry. Give yourself a few weeks to find your feet, then think about when she's feeding.

IF ONLY SOMEONE HAD TOLD ME: ADVICE FROM PARENTS

- Too much milk in one go without a burp = copious milky vomit down your top.
- Changing a baby's milk turns number twos a funny colour.
- Babies go from quite happy to desperately hungry in the blink of an eye. One minute you're quite happily playing building blocks; the next you're sprinting to the kitchen for a bottle or whipping out a breast. They love to keep you on your toes.
- If breastfeeding, don't leave the house without breast pads. Milk running down the front of your t-shirt in the supermarket isn't a great look.
- There's no point cutting a baby off mid-feed to answer the phone or a knock at the door because the person on the phone or at the door won't hear a word you say over the screams of outrage from your baby.
- Think you've got your baby clean in the bath? Think again. Wait until she puts her read right back and you see what's in the folds under her chin. Mmm. Four-day-old milky cheese stuff.

6. Befriending other parents

You've no doubt got all sorts of friends you've made at different stages in your life – at school, at college or university, in various jobs, at the gym and so on. Friendship is based on a mutual interest, having something in common, and now that you're a parent you have a whole new focus in life, so why not make some new friends who are on the same page as you? Don't think of them as friends; think of them as sanity savers!

Myth buster. Many dads assume that it's up to Mum to make friends once the baby's born. But the guidance in this chapter applies to dads as much as it does to mums – every parent benefits from knowing other parents, and being able to share their experiences.

Most parents want to make friends with other parents, especially with first babies, who have no siblings for company. There's no better feeling than sitting in the garden with your friend on a hot, sunny afternoon while your partners fire up the barbecue and your children run about shouting and laughing. Moments like that make all the hard work of parenting worthwhile.

KNOWING THE BENEFITS

There's a reason why this chapter falls so early in the book – right after getting through your baby's first six weeks. The sooner you get to know some other parents, the more support you have as you adjust to parenting yourself.

Until you became a mum or dad, you may have been quite happy that you had plenty of friends to turn to, and had no interest whatsoever in making any new ones. But once your baby comes, life changes, and you may feel that you need more friends who have children and live nearby.

Of course, you may already have an army of friends who are parents, and if so, hooray, because they can offer you lots of help and advice. But many new parents also find they like to go out and meet parents in their local area who have babies of a similar age.

Here are some of the benefits of getting to know other parents:

• *Company*: A day can really drag when it's just you and your baby. The four walls at home can close in, and you start to wonder when you last had an intelligent, adult conversation. Getting out and seeing other people helps you avoid feelings of depression and isolation, and your baby loves being around other people just as much as you do.

• *Comparing notes*: Confused about sterilising? Not sure whether your baby has colic or is just grumpy? Convinced your baby's got one leg longer than the other? The mind of the parent is an anxious, exhausting place full of confusion. Other parents are excellent sounding boards, helping you work out your worries and find new ideas and strategies to apply to your parenting.

• *Confidence*: The more time you spend around other parents, the more your confidence grows – partly by learning from others (their mistakes and their triumphs) and partly because everything you do is reinforced and normalised.

• *Laughter*: Parenting is a whole lot easier with a sense of humour. Spending time with friends can really help you see the lighter side of parenting.

• *Practical help*: The more help you have, the better. And when you make friends with other parents, you have people to turn to when you need a hand – someone to watch your baby while you take the dog to the vet, someone to help you assemble Junior's ridiculously complicated baby gym, someone to help you puree five bags of carrots and so on.

• *Sense of self*: It's not all about your baby. In Chapter 11, I talk about keeping a sense of yourself when you're a parent, so you're not just Mum or Dad, you're you, the person you were before you had a baby. Friends help you remember who you are, because while you may talk about babies sometimes, you also have a coffee, go see a film, laugh over a joke, compare notes on the latest Hollywood gossip and so on.

• *Socialisation for your baby*: When I used to meet up with mum friends we would put the babies together on the floor. Often, they just ignored each other and did their own thing, but it was lovely to see when they took an interest in their little friends. It never hurts to have babies get to know other babies – especially because we're talking about first-borns here who don't have other children around them at home.

'My little boy was like a different baby when we went out to baby groups or went to a friend's house for coffee. He would go from whinging and whining at home and refusing to be put down to sunshine and smiles and wriggling about quite happily on the floor when we were out. At first I got upset about it – I thought he didn't like me much, and so was only happy when he was with other people. Then a friend pointed out that he was probably just more relaxed at her house because I was more relaxed. I realised she was right – I was getting fed up and lonely at home. I'd been working full-time in an office for eight years, and now I was sitting at home every day on maternity leave. I've always been a sociable sort, and I guess Rory is the same. From then on I made sure we went out every day, even if just to the park.'
Jemima, mum to Rory

COUNTING ON BOTH NOVICE AND EXPERIENCED PARENTS
You know best what kind of people you get on with, but when thinking about which parents you include in your support network, I advise thinking about three types of parent:

- *Parents with babies around the same age as yours*: You have a lot in common, and can learn together. And the great benefit is that if your friendship goes the distance, your children are of a similar age and so play nicely together (well, you hope so!).
- *Parents with slightly older children*: There's something to be said for also getting to know parents with young children, but whose children are older than yours (or a mum whose first-born is older than yours, but whose second-born is the same age, for example). These parents have a bit more experience, and can offer you some useful guidance; and babies and toddlers enjoy being around children who are a bit older.
- *Parents with teenage and/or grown-up children*: Don't discount older parents who've been there, done that, got the t-shirt. They have a wealth of knowledge and experience that you can benefit from.

'Having kids has helped us meet so many new people, and if you're open to people helping, there's a lot you can learn. We made good friends with families with children of similar ages, but I was surprised to find it easier as well to get on with older parents. There's this sense of "wow, you did it" when you talk to them, but they're usually happy to admit they got plenty wrong along the way!'
Zach, dad to Alison and Jonathan

TRYING DIFFERENT WAYS TO MEET OTHER MUMS AND DADS
Making new friends can feel like a daunting task. But there are loads of different ways to get to know other parents, and they don't have to push you out of your comfort zone.

Attending baby groups and classes
This is probably the most popular, and the easiest, way to meet other parents – especially those with babies around the same age.

You may be invited to an antenatal group by your midwife or health visitor, and you can find out about parent-and-baby groups in the area (often the National Childbirth Trust (NCT) runs several). There are also specific groups, such as for young mums, for parents of twins or triplets, and for breastfeeding mums.

Then you have a choice of classes, and depending on where you live, there might be quite a range. Baby massage, bounce and rhyme, swimming classes – you're bound to find something that interests you.

Tip: Your local children's centre, the library, local parenting magazines and noticeboards in community centres, churches and supermarkets often have listings for classes and groups. And if you can't find a group that interests you, start your own!

Browsing the internet

Okay, making friends online feels a bit like internet dating, but I've made some of my best mummy friends this way, and I know countless others who have as well. It works like this: you join a parenting website that has an online forum or message board in which you can get to know other parents. You chat for a bit online or via email. If the parent friend lives far away from you, you may simply carry on in this way – being modern-day pen pals. If the parent lives near you, you can set up a meeting and take it from there.

It was when George was six weeks old that I first stumbled across the Netmums website (www.netmums.co.uk). On the 'Meet a Mum' board I found lots of other new mums who were looking to make new friends. I emailed some of them, and we got chatting via email. It was all a bit strange – reading their emails and trying to work out whether we would get on, and knowing they were doing the same.

Some mummies I didn't meet up with; I didn't think we had enough in common. But others I hit it off with. I met up with a couple individually, which was nerve-wracking at first but then a lot of fun (I recall one of their husbands continually ringing to check on his wife in case I was a nutcase). And then one mummy

I was emailing realised that there was a group of us all emailing each other and suggested we meet up. We did, and our little group of six mummies and six babies was established. The Netmums, as I call them, and I are still friends to this day.

So, you can use the internet to make new friends, if you're prepared to get past the awkwardness. Of course, the usual safety rule applies – meet a prospective friend in a public place. Neutral territory makes the first meeting easier in any case.

Tip: Parenting forums aren't just about making friends. You can use them to get information and parents' input on a wide range of subjects. For example, you can read what other parents say about feeding and sleep and illness; and you can post your own questions. Many forums also have a section called something like 'Having a Bad Day' in which you can have a rant or share your feelings on a grey and dreary afternoon, and other parents will give you a virtual hug and some positive encouragement.

Going out and about

Random strangers can become good friends. Don't get me wrong; I'm not suggesting you just march up to any parent you quite like the look of in the street and demand, 'Wanna be my friend?' That's going to get you nowhere (other than ridiculed). But when you're out somewhere with other parents, if you find yourself striking up a conversation with one and getting on well, perhaps suggest a coffee sometime or a 'play date'.

> 'I met Jane at the park. I used to take Carly every Friday afternoon, and I began to recognise another mummy as being there each week. We started smiling at each other and nodding hello, then one day I was pushing Carly on the swings when Jane came over and put her little boy in the next-door swing. We got to chatting, and I suggested a brew at the cafe in the park. Since then, we've become good friends. In fact, Jane was my bridesmaid at my wedding last year.'
> Natalie, mum to Carly and Max

WELCOME TO THE WORLD OF PARENT AND BABY GATHERINGS

For the uninitiated, parent and baby gatherings can be quite an experience. A whole roomful of chatting parents, many tired and emotional, and babies ranging from the peaceful slumberer to the ear-shattering wailer can feel a bit overwhelming. I remember within five minutes of my first mummy and baby group George did his most spectacular poo yet, which necessitated a total strip and scrub down, and by the time I finished (having worked my way through all my wipes and several other mothers' as well) I was Stressed with a capital S – I hadn't quite mastered clean-ups yet, and I convinced myself every mum there was watching me and tutting.

The good news is, in no time at all, you feel right at home around other parents and babies. But until then here's the lowdown on what to expect.

Tip: Give a parent and baby group three visits before you decide it's not for you. At first, you may feel uncomfortable, but as you get to know people you may find you enjoy it.

Spending time with other people's babies

Babies can be loud and stinky and sticky and grumpy and grabby. You knew that of course thanks to your little one. But you love your baby, which means you're pretty immune to his eau-de-dirty-nappy and drooly kisses. Other people's babies, however, may be a little less delightful at times.

Don't worry if you find yourself not adoring all the babies you meet. Being a mum or a dad doesn't mean you have to go mushy over every baby in the world – just yours.

You may find yourself feeling hugely protective over your little one as you watch him try to hold his own among his peers. A baby taps him on the head with his rattle, another crawls right over him, and another drools fetchingly all over Junior's favourite teddy. Alright, it's not ideal – but keep it in perspective, and remember that your baby has to learn to be around others (and to be around germs!).

Telling the truth?

It takes a certain amount of courage to admit to what you worry another parent may see as a failing in you or your baby (though of course it never is). For example, ask a mum how her baby's sleeping at night, and she might respond with, 'Oh, fabulous. Millicent has slept through every night from birth, don't you know. She sleeps 16 hours a night.' Now perhaps this mum does have a miracle child who just loves sleep, but it's more likely that she's either feeling competitive (see the next section) or doesn't feel able to tell the truth because she's uncomfortable admitting how she feels. The best response, in my experience, is just to beam back and say warmly, 'Great. How lovely for you.'

Also consider how open you want to be about how you feel. At first in a parent and baby gathering you may feel more comfortable not telling people much about how you're coping as a parent, but as time goes on and you get to know people, you come to that point where perhaps you're ready to share when you're having a bad day, and get some moral support from your new friends.

'When Christopher was wee my partner and I struggled. He had colic badly, and then he kept getting chest infections so was grumpy and clingy. My wife and I were so fed up, and it felt like everything was falling apart. One day at work I was in a meeting and an important client asked how fatherhood was treating me. I spun a massive lie about how wonderful it all was. I got quite carried away, and ended up saying that Christopher was really advanced for his age and was already saying 'Dada' when he saw me. The client – a dad himself – looked a bit surprised but just smiled. Months later when Christopher finally did start talking I realised how ridiculous I'd been to say he had been talking at six months!'
Martin, dad to Christopher

Stepping out of the parenting race

Parents can be competitive. When did your baby first smile? Mine did it at four weeks. When did your baby start weaning? Mine's started already. When did your baby first roll over? Mine did it at five months. How are you educating your child? You're not?! But she's six months old – I'd already run Henry though the major Latin verbs by that age...

Most parents are happy to accept babies just as they are – and they understand that all babies are different, and progress at their own speed. But you do meet the odd parent who seems to view child-rearing as some kind of race or competition.

George, bless him, was a content little baby who was quite happy to just lie about and watch the world go by. Consequently, he showed little interest in rolling or sitting or crawling for some time. Occasionally, I'd meet a mum who'd seem to think that George was backwards compared to her baby. It frustrated me, but eventually I came to realise that these were insecure mums if they needed to compare their babies, and I could just ignore their comments.

Letting go of judgement

I recall being at a mum and baby group once when the group leader announced that someone had donated a load of baby jars they had no need of, and if anyone wanted them to let her know – but, she concluded, she was sure that no one in the room wanted baby jars, because of course our babies were all fed on entirely organic, home-grown and home-cooked meals. I think it was meant to be a joke (though no one laughed), but I didn't appreciate it as it felt like a jibe that any parent in the room who ever fed baby from a jar was in some way an inferior parent.

If you're getting out and about and attending baby groups and classes, you meet all sorts of parents – from the laissez-faire to the super-in-control, and everyone in between (flick to Chapter 1 for more info on parenting styles). Some you'll get on with; some you won't. But whatever parents you meet, your best approach is to view them with compassion and without judgement – we're all just parents doing our best in a difficult job.

> 'I'm not an "earth mummy". I didn't breastfeed, I bottle fed. I gave them dummies (and they still have them at night). I use disposable nappies. I weaned them early, mainly on jars. I did controlled crying. I put them in nursery from a young age. I have good reasons for all my decisions as a mum, but still I found myself feeling bad inside when I went to one particular baby group, like the women were looking down their noses at me. But you know what? My girls have always been so happy, so I reckon I must have done something right!'
> Melissa, mum to Anna and Bella

STRENGTHENING TIES TO THOSE ALREADY IN YOUR LIFE

This chapter is all about making new friends, but it would be incomplete without a section on thinking about who's already in your life who can offer you friendship and support. Think about your friends and family and colleagues and acquaintances – who has children? Whom could you turn to with questions, or to offer some comfort and help?

As I explain in Chapter 1, you can parent as you want to parent – you don't have to be influenced by anyone else's opinion or experiences. But letting other people in now again can help you feel less alone, and a happier, more confident parent.

IF ONLY SOMEONE HAD TOLD ME: ADVICE FROM PARENTS

- New parents can be a bit bonkers. So don't judge people too quickly!
- Parent friends are the ones with whom you can share the 'dark side' of you as a parent ('I hate babies!' 'I miss my old life!' 'I gave up my career for this!') on a bad day, and they

won't judge you, and they'll know that while there's a little truth to what you say, you don't really mean it as it sounds.
•   Who else will talk quite happily about poo with you?
•   The best thing about getting out and meeting other parents? They coo over your baby.

7. Weaning: food, glorious food!

A baby's first year is a year of two halves: birth to six months – milk; six months to age one – solids. Breast, bottle, formula, puree, finger foods – the journey can feel a bit daunting. Don't worry, all babies get there in the end.

Weaning has to be my favourite part of parenting in the first year. The expression on George's face the first time I popped in a spoonful of baby rice – pure wonder! Seeing George exploring different foods for himself was amazing and staggeringly messy.

In this chapter, I take you through the weaning process, so you can coast through meal times and enjoy watching your baby progress from milk-sipper to muncher extraordinaire.

FROM PUREE TO SOLIDS

It's frustrating – no sooner have you got the hang of milk feeding, and probably by now fallen into something of a routine, than you have to shake things up by teaching your baby to eat. When you first start weaning, it can feel like a long gap between that first taste of food through to your baby feeding herself the same food you eat. But in fact, it's a really fun journey and an opportunity to get to know more about your baby's personality.

Your mission between six months (or four/five months if you wean early) and a year is to help your baby progress from eating purees to a variety of solid foods, and from eating just a little to eating three meals plus snacks each day. So, you gradually decrease the amount of milk you offer and increase meals, and you broaden the range of flavours and increase the lumpiness of the foods as you go.

You usually start with pureed fruits and vegetables, and baby rice mixed with your baby's milk. Once your baby's gobbling that down, you can progress to introducing the other food groups – dairy, meat/fish and carbs, all pureed up. As your baby gets older, you make the puree a little lumpier and you start to offer finger foods, until by her first birthday she's off the mush and starting to eat more like a toddler.

Tip: Invest in a hand blender, which allows you to whizz up solid food into purees in seconds.

There are a few foods to avoid in your baby's first year:
• Cow's milk.
• Foods she can choke on (for example whole cherry to-matoes and whole grapes – cut them into small pieces).
• Foods that may contain harmful bacteria (pretty much the same list as you avoid while pregnant, for example soft cheeses, pâté and undercooked or raw eggs, but also avoid honey).
• Low-fat foods.
• Salt and sugar.
• Shark, swordfish and marlin (they contain mercury).

TO JAR OR NOT TO JAR?

I was all set for home-cooking George's meals (which was a pretty brave undertaking as I am notorious among friends and family for my woefully lacking culinary skills). Problem 1: George didn't seem impressed by my efforts. Problem 2: George fell ill at seven months and we were stuck in a hospital for weeks which couldn't provide baby meals. The result? Jars.

At first, I felt like I was a Bad Mummy for using jars. Then I looked around and realised a lot of other mums use them, and if you look at the ingredients on them, many of them are actually good options. I tried to incorporate home-cooked food when I could (not exactly possible while living in a children's ward), but we used jars until George turned one. And he loved them!

The cons are that they can work out expensive, and they can be pretty bland, which can make baby a bit resistant to lumpy, flavourful food down the road. But mixed in with some home-made food, I think they do no harm – and they're very useful for when you're out and about.

BABY-LED WEANING

For years mums and dads have been spooning gloop into babies' mouths until they develop the knack of holding the spoon themselves and getting it in their mouth (as opposed to their eyes/ears/hair). Then along came a group of parents who suggested that babies can learn to feed themselves without your intervention, and there's no need for all this pureeing and spoon-feeding.

The idea of baby-led weaning is this: from six months of age (not before) you put your baby in her highchair and give her a selection of finger foods to try. For example, to start with you may offer a rusk and a stick of cooked carrot. Then, as your baby gets older and gets the hang of eating, you can offer a greater variety of foods, such as sandwiches and pasta. Eventually, your baby will be happy to use a spoon to eat foods other than finger food, such as yoghurt.

Baby-led weaning has a lot going for it. It allows your baby independence, and it frees you up from standing over her and trying to get her to eat. And advocates of the approach say it leads to babies who are less fussy in their eating and more willing to try new foods.

The downside is that your baby usually doesn't eat a lot at first, until she gets the hang of feeding herself, so she probably still wants a fair amount of milk. And you may worry about choking, but as long as your baby is sitting upright and you stay with her, she should be sufficiently developed by this age to handle the food in her mouth.

You meet some parents who follow baby-led weaning religiously, and never spoon-feed their babies. But many parents combine the approach with a touch of spoon-feeding. For example, a six-month-old baby rather enjoys some mashed banana for dessert, but isn't able to get the spoon in the bowl, the banana on the spoon and the spoon in her mouth. So you can hand her the spoon, and then guide her.

'So messy. Mush where you wouldn't believe mush could end up. Funny smells emanating from nooks and crannies where peas, chunks of potato and grated cheese have accumulated. But so much fun! It was like Peter and me, little chums, munching away together. Some of our best laughs were when he started eating with us. Spaghetti is the best. Probably easiest serving it in the bath.'
Simon, dad to Peter

EATING TOGETHER AS A FAMILY

'The family that eats together, stays together,' so they say. It's never too early to introduce family mealtimes, though of course it's not always possible when Mum and/or Dad are working.

The more you can sit your baby at the table with you while you eat, the more she learns about how to eat, and the social side of eating together. You may be surprised just what your baby's willing to try when she sees her parents tucking in.

When George was first weaning I fed him in his highchair in the kitchen. He'd eat a bit, then get bored. I'd try to coax him to eat some more. He'd throw a breadstick at me. Then I decided to have a go at eating tea with him. I cooked dinner and George and I would sit together and get started, then my husband would join us when he came in. We saw a real difference in George from then on; he was much more interested in his food.

Tip: Even if you only sit down together once a week as a family for a meal, that helps.

'Since Charlotte was a newborn I'd often have her on my lap while eating – she's so clingy it's easier that way than having her scream the place down. When she was six months one day she just grabbed a chip off my plate and tucked in. Later, she got another one and tried to feed it to

me. It was lovely, feeling she was a part of our mealtime like that.'
Claire, mum to Charlotte and James

A NOTE ON MESS
No chapter on weaning would be complete without thinking about mess. Apple sauce in eyebrows, in hair, in armpits, between toes; pureed cottage pie up the curtains, on the bookshelf, on the cat. Weaning is a hugely messy business!

Babies don't give a fig about mess, and nor should they – they need to explore more than just the taste of food, but also its texture, how it feels in their chubby fists. They need to practise eating for themselves, so they learn how to self-feed. And yes, they need to try out their throwing arm.

Getting wound up about mess achieves nothing but making you (and possibly the baby) unhappy. Okay, it's a drag cleaning up, and sometimes you have your work cut out for you getting fish pie out of your baby's hair, but it's all fixable. And if you don't want to get splattered with tomato pasta, stay beyond the five-metre exclusion zone around your baby's highchair.

IF ONLY SOMEONE HAD TOLD ME: ADVICE FROM PARENTS
•   When feeding a baby spag bol, move the highchair to the middle of the room, well away from the cream-painted walls (better yet, do it in the garden).
•   You might not think cheese toastie dipped in yogurt or rusk with pea puree is gourmet cuisine, but your baby does – let her experiment with flavours.
•   Buy bibs. Many bibs.
•   Feed your child anything orange coloured and see it on their clothes for eternity.
•   Put your child in her best outfit and it will be a mess in five minutes. Put her in scruffy clothes and she will stay pristine.

- Baby food can be delicious. You may find yourself joining your baby in her supper!
- Babies pull interesting faces when given a new flavour, especially a sharp one – have your mobile phone video camera ready and you may earn a few bob on *You've Been Framed*.

8. Sleep is everything

Ask a parent the hardest thing about having a baby and it's a safe bet their answer will be 'exhaustion'. By day, babies are such lovely, cuddly, cute little creatures that make your heart melt; by night they're lovely, cuddly, cute little creatures that make you very, very tired.

When it comes to struggling with sleep deprivation, I have abundant sympathy for parents. If I think back to George's early weeks, I remember cold, dark winter nights, trying to stay awake during feeds that seemed to go on for hours, staring into the silent darkness and feeling like I was the only person awake at this ungodly hour. My son, George, didn't sleep through the night until he was 18 months, and it wasn't until he was approaching two and a half that he consistently slept well. I was a tired mummy for a good couple of years.

Sleep, for parents, is everything. Sleep well and you handle colic and feeding and illness and the myriad other issues that arise with your baby in the day. Sleep badly for a prolonged period and parenting can become a real struggle.

In this chapter I take you through some of the basics of sleep, so both you and your baby can get the shut-eye you need to be happy and healthy, to start the day with a smile, rather than a groan.

A NOTE ON SAFE SLEEPING FOR BABIES
Before we dive in to thinking about how you and your baby can sleep well, there's some information you need to consider about Junior's safety while asleep.

I hope you've heard it all before, but in case not, here's an overview of safety considerations for slumbering infants to avoid the risk of accidents and sudden infant death syndrome (SIDS):
- Cot bars should be between 45 and 65 millimetres apart.

- Don't use a pillow or duvet under the age of one.
- Ensure the cot mattress fits the cot snugly (ideally, buy a new mattress).
- Keep the room not too cold and not too hot (between 16 and 20 degrees) and don't bundle your baby in too many covers (if you're unsure whether your baby's too hot, put your finger down the back of his neck – if he's hot and sweaty there, remove some layers).
- Only use the highest setting of the cot until Junior is rolling over, and then drop it down.
- Put your baby to sleep on his back.
- Remember 'feet to foot': put your baby's feet at the bottom of the cot so he can't wriggle under the covers.

Guidance from a support organisation: National Childbirth Trust

NCT is the UK's largest charity for parents, supporting thousands of parents-to-be and parents of young children every year. NCT's website (www.nct.org.uk) includes lots of information and support on all aspects of pregnancy, birth and life with a new baby, including information on safe co-sleeping. Sleeping in the same bed as your baby, called co-sleeping or bed-sharing, can help maintain breastfeeding at night and reduce sleep disruption for mothers, fathers and babies. Around half of all UK mothers sleep with their baby in bed at some time.

The Department of Health advises that bed-sharing should be avoided if one or both parents is a smoker; has consumed alcohol; has taken any drugs, prescription or otherwise, that affect perception, cause drowsiness or affect depth of sleep; or is excessively tired so that they might not be able to respond to the baby.

If you do decide to co-sleep, you need to:
- Make sure your baby can't fall out of bed, either by putting a rail at the side, or by pushing the bed up against the wall.

• Keep your baby cool by using sheets and blankets rather than a duvet.
• Always put your baby to sleep on his back rather than his front or side.
• Don't use a pillow – babies don't need a pillow until they are a year old.
• Never risk falling asleep with your baby on a sofa or armchair.

KNOWING HOW BABIES SLEEP

It may not seem it when you've bags under bags under bags under your eyes, but babies sleep a lot. A newborn sleeps for around 18 hours a day, and around 15 hours by month three. In the daytime, this inability to stay awake for long is rather nice – you get nice milky, snoozy cuddles after feeds, and you get to put the baby down and get stuff done around the house. But at night-time your baby's two-hourly or so waking is pretty wearing.

The problem is simple: your baby's sleep cycle is much shorter than yours. An adult usually has between six and nine hours sleep a night; a new baby usually sleeps for between one and four hours at most before waking. In addition, a baby spends more time in dream sleep (rapid eye movement, or REM sleep) than an adult, which means he's in a light sleep and easily disturbed.

As babies grow, they cut back on daytime sleep, consolidating it into naps, and sleep for longer periods at night (hooray!). Every baby is different, however, and while you can read all kinds of stuff about what your baby 'should' be doing by x months, I think that really there's no such thing as 'normal'. For example your baby may:

• Have three long naps a day and then sleep for 12 hours at night.
• Refuse to nap in the day and sleep for 14 hours at night.
• Sleep well at nap times, but struggle to fall asleep in the evening.

- Sleep well, but get you up three times a night just for a quick cuddle.
- Refuse to settle for naps or at bedtime, but sleep through once down.
- Get you up every three hours or so every night.
- Sleep through from six weeks.

And hundreds of other variations. I have friends whose babies took four-hour naps right through to the age of one and still slept beautifully at night, and I have friends who, like me, were pacing nurseries with bright-eyed babies in the early hours for month after month. The point is: whatever you're baby's doing, don't worry about it. Your baby will settle in time. (And if you think, as did I, that your baby's the worst sleeper of anyone's you know, console yourself with the idea that while other mums and dads may be finding sleep a doddle, they're probably going to encounter problems in another area of child-rearing that your baby sails on through.)

Tip: The phrase 'sleeping through' crops up often between parents of young babies. If your baby's still getting you up at night, it can be pretty depressing to talk to a 'perfect' mum (more on these in Chapter 6) who says hers has slept through from birth. Make sure you've understood that mum's definition of 'sleeping through' before you get too despondent. Some parents use it to mean sleeping from bedtime until morning, say 7 p.m. to 7 a.m.; others use it to mean sleeping between midnight and 5 a.m.

UNDERSTANDING THE EFFECTS OF SLEEP DEPRIVATION

There's a reason why sleep deprivation has been used throughout history as an interrogation/torture tactic. Being exhausted sucks. No one likes feeling tired; the body just isn't designed to go without sleep for long. Sleep is essential for a healthy body. That's why you can't go long without sleep before feeling ill and losing the plot (in case you're interested, the longest anyone has gone without sleep, in a scientifically validated study, is eleven days, and the young lad was delusional by day four).

Disturbed or absent sleep that continues for a prolonged period has the following effects on you:

- *Cognitive function*: You may be more forgetful, find it harder to concentrate and do daft things like put the car in gear and try to drive off without having switched on the engine.
- *Health*: You may suffer from aching muscles and headaches and find it hard to get warm. You may also find you get rundown, and come down with every cold and cough that Junior passes to you.
- *Mood*: You may feel down and negative, depressed even, and you may be irritable. Hell hath no fury like a parent exhausted.
- *Tiredness-induced behaviours*: A lot of tired parents report either losing weight through not bothering to eat or gaining weight through comfort eating. You may smoke more, drink more, exercise more or less – all ways of coping with the low mood brought on by exhaustion.

Not very cheery reading, I know. But by understanding sleep deprivation, you realise that it's important to do what you can to sleep better, because happy parent equals happy baby. I offer some suggestions later in this chapter for how you can encourage baby to sleep better, and how you can alleviate your own tiredness.

Another benefit of being aware of how sleep deprivation affects you is that if you find yourself struggling to focus in the day, or constantly heading to the doctor's with ailments, or snapping at your partner and getting tearful, or chomping biscuits from dawn till dusk – now you can see the reason. There's little point doing Sudoku to sharpen your mind, taking a weird combination of herbs to build up your body, worrying that you're clinically depressed or going on a one-bowl-of-seaweed-a-day diet if all that's wrong is that you're tired. Treat the root cause, not the symptom of the problem. Find a way to be less exhausted, and see whether the other problems in your life disappear as a result.

'I remember being in the ward with Eloise the night after I gave birth, and the woman opposite me called for the nurse and demanded a sedative because she couldn't sleep what with all the noise from the babies (in fact, hers was the loudest). I wasn't surprised when the nurse turned her down, but I knew how that exhausted woman felt!'
Bonnie, mum to Eloise

'It became a running joke in my office the daft things I did after Lisa was born. Like turning up in odd socks. And stapling an invoice to my tie. And spilling a cup of coffee all over my computer. I was a zombie for a while. Good job it wasn't appraisal time!'
Andy, dad to Lisa

Tip: Keep in mind that the season affects your ability to cope with sleep deprivation and disturbance. In summer we generally sleep a little less, and we find it easier to wake up in the morning. In the depths of winter even 7 a.m. can feel too early, and we feel more tired and want to sleep for longer. So if your baby is born in the autumn or winter and you're finding night feeds a real drag, look forward to the lighter months – not only will your baby be more settled, but an evening and early morning feed will be in the light, much easier to manage. Oh, and if you're up in the night over the winter, set the heating to come on at some point. Getting out of bed to go to a baby is hard enough without having to creep through an icy house.

TRYING DIFFERENT STRATEGIES TO IMPROVE SLEEP
I could write an entire book (as have others) on methods you can try to help your baby sleep. The following sections give you some ideas you can try – all tried and tested and thumbs-upped by myself and/or parents I know.

Filling that tummy

Many babies wake at night because they're hungry. A milk feed and they settle right back to sleep. If your baby just won't settle, it may be that hunger's the culprit.

Tip: Don't cut out night feeds too soon. Yes, you don't want to get up in the night, or stay up late to do a final pre-bed feed, but if your baby needs the milk, you'll have a miserable night going back and forth to him. Sometimes a drink of milk is all it takes to settle the baby.

If your baby is under six months old and has an insatiable appetite, you may consider weaning him a little early and introducing some food to fill that tummy before bed. Head to Chapter 7 for the lowdown on weaning.

> 'I used to like giving George a sleepy feed right before I went to bed at about 11 p.m., because I knew once he'd finished and I put him down I could get in bed and SLEEP without being woken for a decent stretch.'
> Ally, dad to George

Considering where baby sleeps

Experts recommend that your baby sleeps in the same room as his parents for the first six months. After six months, you may decide to move baby into his own room – and many parents find that this helps the baby (and Mum and Dad) sleep better, because they're not waking each other with their night-time noises.

Tip: When moving your baby into a new room, do so gradually. Try putting your baby down for naps in there at first, before progressing to night-time. And if the move to his own room coincides with a move from a Moses basket or crib to a cot, try placing the basket or crib top in the cot at first. It can be quite unsettling for a baby used to being in a cosy little basket or crib to then be placed in a vast cot.

Some parents prefer to co-sleep with their baby (have baby in bed with them). This is great for bonding, and you may find that bringing your baby into bed with you – either permanently, or because he's really unsettled or ill – ensures a better night's sleep for all. But make sure you check out the safety information on this: basically, remove any risk that your baby can suffocate under the covers or be rolled upon by a parent, and ensure he won't overheat. See pages 110–11 for the NCT guidelines on this.

Establishing a wind-down routine

From about six weeks you can start devising a bedtime routine for your baby. Each day that goes by, your baby becomes more familiar with what the routine signifies: calming down, and then sleep. The routine becomes a comfort as they grow; my little boy George still has the same routine at age three, and he loves it.

You can set up any routine you like, but most parents incorporate some or all of the following in the half hour or so before lights out:

- Warm bath.
- Massage.
- Into pyjamas.
- Read a story.
- Cuddle and milk.
- Lullaby.
- Night night words (George's got extended over the years and are now: 'Nighty night, sweetheart. Sleep tight. Sweet dreams. I love you. See you in the morning when the sun is up. Thanks for being a good boy today. I'll check on you later and give you a kiss and cuddle when you're sleeping.' If I don't say it verbatim he corrects me!)

The golden rule with bedtime routines is to keep everything quiet and calm. A tickle after the bath gets the baby all excited, as does a rousing, top-of-the-lungs rendition of 'Wheels on the Bus' once he's tucked up in bed.

Tip: Develop a 'night-time voice' to use with your baby – a soft tone you use at bedtime and during the night. Make it pretty boring and non-emotive, to signal to your baby that this isn't a time for interaction and play.

'I established a routine with my first baby, Oliver, and I found my husband and I enjoyed it as much as him, so when the next baby came along, we did the same pretty much from birth. The best thing I've found about having a routine is that if someone comes to babysit, they can follow the routine and the baby knows what to expect, and when we go away with the children they've always settled well. I think the routine makes them feel safe and secure. You have to take your time with it though – they seem to sense if you're rushing through to catch the start of *EastEnders*!'
Tracy, mum to Oliver and Jacob

Timing naps, bedtime and getting up?

In Chapter 1, I talk about parenting styles and how you need to find your own way of being a mum and dad – there are no rules. Some parents and babies thrive on routine; some prefer to just go with the flow. Most parents sit somewhere between the two extremes of running the baby's life to a timetable with military precision and floating through the day and night with no structure at all.

Tip: With a newborn baby, don't tie yourself up in knots trying to create a rigid sleep routine. Your baby hasn't a clue what you're trying to do, and will sleep and wake whenever he pleases. Agonising over nap times and bedtime and when you start your day only stresses you (and your baby) out.

As your baby gets older, you may start to see patterns emerge in the timing of daytime naps, and you can go with these. Bedtime is often set by parents – most parents I know opt for between 7 p.m. and 8.30 p.m. – keeping a baby up late is a recipe for a tired and fractious infant. As for getting-up time, well, that's hard to control. Some babies are up and at 'em at 5 a.m.; some will take a feed between 4 a.m. and 7 a.m. and then nod off again; some babies just snooze on through till breakfast time.

'I remember in the early days we just kept Louise with us all the time – so we'd watch TV until 11 at night and leave her in her Moses sleeping or watching the lights on the tele. Then we'd wonder why we couldn't get her to settle when we went to bed – she'd cry and cry. Eventually it dawned on me she was over-tired – she needed to have a bedtime!'
Beth, mum to Louise

Thinking about sleep associations

How does your baby like to fall asleep? In your arms? Sucking Mum's breast or a bottle? Being rocked on a rocking chair? On Dad's shoulder?

The phrase 'by any means necessary' often came to me when George was a baby. In the early months I did whatever I could to get him to sleep – and some nights that meant me spending a long time in his nursery, feeding him until he was sleeping, then waiting and waiting until I thought it might be safe to lay him down.

Eventually, I came to realise that George had picked up some habits – he preferred to go to sleep in my arms, sucking away. Such a lovely way to go to sleep; I quite understood. But it took some time to encourage George to go down in his cot awake and soothe himself to sleep, rather than monopolise me as sleeping facilitator for a good hour each night.

When babies are tiny, I think you have to just go with your baby. But as he gets older you may start to realise that your baby's dependent on something you do to get to sleep – which means when he wakes up in the night, he can't go back to sleep by himself. What you need to do is try to help your baby learn to 'self-soothe', which means find comfort without you sufficient to fall asleep. The baby can't always fall sleep on you, or sucking away; so at some point he has to learn to sleep by himself. The only way forward is to give him a lovely cuddle and milk feed, but put him down before he falls asleep. He won't like it much at first, but you can extend the bedtime routine to staying with him for a little while, perhaps stroking his tummy and singing songs, and then you say 'night night' firmly and leave the room.

Blocking out noise

Myth buster. Babies don't need quiet to sleep! You don't need to tiptoe around your home once baby's asleep – if baby gets used to sleeping amid silence all the time, he's going to wake up at the slightest noise. But if you start to wonder whether baby's sensitive to noise, and is getting disturbed during naps or in the evening, try playing white noise in or outside the room – you can buy CDs. I bought a fabulous lullaby maker for George that had rain and waves noise options, and he used to nod off nicely to that.

Blacking out the room

Most parents find that blackout blinds or curtains help a baby sleep, especially during nap times and during the early evening and early morning in the summer months. But the blackness in the baby's room can be a bit much (if you've ever stumbled into the nursery half asleep in the middle of the night and stubbed your toe on the cot because it's that dark you haven't a clue where you're going, you'll know what I mean). A little plug-in night-light in the corner helps; and you may also invest in a light-show that plays on the ceiling for a while after you say night-night (so you don't plunge your baby straight into the dark).

Tip: When it comes to night feeds, the less light you're able to feed by, the better. If you put the big overhead light on to feed by, your baby will wake right up and be harder to soothe back to sleep. Try a dimmer switch, or a very low watt lamp – you can get lamps that dim right down).

Snuggling in sleepwear

Is your baby struggling to sleep because he's too hot, or too cold, or twisted up in his bedding? It's worth investigating whether baby's comfortable enough at night.

Tiny babies often sleep better when swaddled – wrapped up nice and snug in a blanket, which makes them feel embraced tightly as they were in the womb. There's a knack to swaddling, and you may find it useful to ask a parent who knows how to show you. Here's a basic guide:

1. Lay a swaddling blanket or baby sheet out, and fold down a corner, then lie your baby on his back so that the back of his neck is on the fold. (Warning: don't use a thick blanket or your baby may get too hot.)
2. Take the left corner of the blanket and bring it across your baby, tucking the material under him (not so tightly that he can't move).
3. Take the bottom corner of the blanket and bring it up to his left shoulder.
4. Take the remaining right corner of the blanket and wrap it over him, so that he's a snug little package.

Older babies seem to get on well with baby sleeping bags, which ensure they don't get in a fangle or kick off their blanket.

Ditching dummies?

Some babies just love their dummies. George was certainly an addict. The problem was, every time he woke up and realised he'd lost his dummy, he shouted until my husband or I staggered into the room and popped it back in. This went on for months and was pretty exhausting. The plus side was that it was quick and easy to settle George at night – all he wanted was his dummy. The down side was that we were up and down like yoyos because every time he fell asleep the dummy fell out of his mouth.

You may reach a point where you decide the dummy's going in the bin. Yes, you have a few days of hard work on your hands as your baby protests the loss of his lovely sucky comfort; but then he kicks the habit and learns to sleep without the dummy.

'My wife and I got so sick of getting up to give Thomas his dummy at night that one bedtime we just chucked the whole stash in there, about ten I think. And we didn't get up that night! The next evening we watched him on the video baby monitor. Clever chap was finding them himself.'

Aled, dad to Thomas

Crying it out

Surely one of the most debated topics among parents! When you've tried everything you can think of to encourage your baby to sleep better, do you leave him to cry?

The thinking behind crying it out is that if you know that an older baby (some say three months plus, some say six) isn't ill or scared or cold or hungry and is just crying because he wants to see you, by leaving him to settle himself you break this habit and teach him to self-soothe. There are all kinds of variations on this approach, from not going to your baby at all and leaving him to cry and cry, to going in at first and then returning after increasing intervals for quick reassurance.

Some parents have firm views either way on the crying-it-out method. Here are some things to consider when deciding whether to use this form of sleep training:

• Tiny babies need attention – they're not cognitively developed enough to learn the lesson of the crying-it-out sleep training method. Leave a young baby to cry on and on and he simply feels abandoned, which isn't ideal for his development. That's why experts only recommend the crying-it-out approach for older babies.

• If leaving your baby to cry, be very sure that there's nothing wrong with him – he's not hot or cold, he's not in pain or running a fever, he's not hungry, he's not wet or soiled, he's not got his foot wedged through the cot bars.

• Don't use the crying-it-out method off and on – either use it, or don't. Otherwise you drag out the process, and weaken its effect because the baby learns that eventually you'll cave and come to him. If you're going to leave your baby to cry, be consistent in your approach or he goes through all that heartache for nothing (see the following section on consistency).

Tip: Whatever your approach to your baby's sleep, try to resist the urge to leap out of bed the moment you hear the beginning of a cry. As my aunt (mum of four) once said to me, the baby starts to feel like he's got you on a piece of string and can get you running to him with just a little tug. Sometimes, if you wait a minute, you find your baby settles himself. In time, you come to know your baby's cries, and you can often tell the difference between a sleepy whimper that will settle and a full-lunged 'Mum-Dad-I've-had-the-most-TERRIFYING-dream-help-me-help-me!' shriek.

Being consistent

As your baby grows up, you find he has an astonishing knack for spotting inconsistencies in your parenting. In our house, George can commonly be heard saying, 'But you said...', to which I reply, 'Oops, yes, silly Mummy.'

Babies are also very tuned in to consistency. Say for three nights when your baby cries you simply go in and say 'Shhh, back to sleep' and then leave his room, but on the fourth night you go in, pick him up and rock him back to sleep. On the fifth night, if you go in and try 'Shhh, back to sleep', your baby will have none of it – he'd much rather have a lovely rocking cuddle, thank you very much.

Now I'm not suggesting that you can't be flexible with your baby and adapt your parenting to his needs. Sometimes you have to break from the norm – for example when your baby is ill or frightened. But there needs to be some kind of norm. Babies are creatures of habit; they like to have some idea of what to expect. So if you're trying to encourage your baby to sleep by himself – without calling for you whenever he stirs – you need to have a level of consistency in your approach, or canny little man that he is, he'll see a weakness and exploit it!

Tip: Work together as parents to come up with a consistent strategy for baby's sleep, and try not to undermine each other.

For example, if Dad is always firm with your baby, doesn't pick him up, but soothes him briefly and firmly while Mum sprints in the moment he murmurs and picks him up for a cuddle, that's pretty confusing for the baby. The result? The baby wants Mum, not Dad, at night! Talk through your ideas, and then try to reach a compromise together.

FINDING A LEVEL OF ACCEPTANCE WITH YOUR BABY'S SLEEP

Go into your local book shop and you'll find a wide range of books on babies and parenting, and each will contain plenty of guidance on how to get your baby to sleep; indeed, there are even entire books dedicated to the subject. A whole range of pro-grammes exist for 'training' babies to sleep, with rules that defeat even the most motivated of parents. The result is a focus on sleep that can push you to a point where Junior's sleeping habits really get you down. I know, I was there.

Here's a controversial idea: accept that your baby doesn't sleep quite as you'd like, but that it won't always be this way.

Now, I'm not suggesting that you don't try different methods to help your baby sleep better (as I suggest in the earlier section 'Trying different strategies to improve sleep'). But I am saying that at a certain level you have to know when to let go and just accept where you are on the sleep front – that dedicating all your energy to 'curing' Junior of his sleep 'problem' may not be doing either of you any good, because it makes you miserable.

> 'The thing with all the advice you hear about sleep is that you apply it, and it might work for a while, but then baby either slips back into the habit, or starts something else. With Lawrence, I would tear my hair out trying to sleep train him, and then I'd think we'd cracked it – he'd sleep well for a week or two – then something else would start up. I spent so much of his first year fixated on getting him to sleep. It made me really tense. Then when Amelie came

along I was more chilled about things. I guess I was more used to getting up in the night then. I don't know if that's what helped, but she settled a lot sooner than Laurie.'
Belinda, mum to Lawrence and Amelie

'I was desperate for my first son to sleep through as he'd often be up in the night for hours at a time, really unsettled! I was a lot more chilled out with my second as I knew the day would finally come where he did sleep through. You seem to get used to having no sleep! I think a good day-time and nighttime routine is essential to get them to get the refreshing sleep they need.'
Maria, mum to Oliver and Thomas

It's not your baby's fault that he doesn't sleep as you'd like. He doesn't have a problem; he just does what comes naturally to him. And though there are plenty of things you can try, and many of them help, you can't control your baby – you can't make him sleep.

The wonderful thing about being a parent is that this little person you create is completely separate to you, and has his own personality and direction in life. One of the skills you develop as a parent is knowing when to step in and guide your child, and when to sit back and accept him as he is. It's not easy to love your child getting you up at 3 a.m. when he's not hungry or wet or cold or ill, but you can accept that he's a little boy who loves his Mummy and Daddy, and loves to cuddle, and there's nothing wrong with that.

The bottom line is this: the sleepless nights won't last forever. Junior will click eventually. Sometimes, babies just need time and patience, and acceptance.

'What drove me mad when Jake was tiny was that I felt like it was just me getting no sleep. Fair enough at first I knew the mums I met at baby groups were tired, but by three months then four then six then nine, and I was still

getting up three or four times a night, I felt so alone with it. It was almost competitive – whose baby slept through first, whose baby slept the most. Jakey just didn't want to sleep much at all, and I got so down about it. Then I realised that there were other mums who got up still as well, but because they weren't getting worried and fed up with it, and thinking their babies should be sleeping better, it wasn't getting to them.'
Sarah, mum to Jake

ALLEVIATING TIREDNESS IN YOURSELF
Parenting is hard enough without adding on layer upon layer of building exhaustion. The more you can do to alleviate tiredness, the better you feel as a parent.

Sleeping when your baby sleeps
So you're looking after your baby on your own, and you're exhausted. Then the baby falls asleep, happily fed and changed and winded, and you reckon he'll be down for a good 45 minutes. You've got dishes to wash, bottles to sterilise, the Sky Planner to set, potatoes to peel for dinner, but boy are you shattered. Stop! Go upstairs, lie down and drift for a while. Domestic tasks don't matter; put yourself first.

One caveat here – baby care experts recommend that you don't fall asleep with your baby in your arms. As lovely and snuggly as it is to creep down the sofa once your baby's nodded off and catch some zzzzs, you may roll and squish him, and the risk of sudden infant death syndrome is raised. Better to put your baby in his cot or basket.

'Everyone told us "Sleep when the baby sleeps". Well that worked for my girlfriend, but not me – I was back at work when the twins were five days old. And shattered. After a couple of days struggling through I decided I'd better kip on my lunch break – so I'd take a quick zizz in the car for

half an hour. Did me the world of good! Attracted some attention from my workmates, but all I cared about was sleep.'
Ian, dad to Henry and Catherine

Parenting in shifts

Okay, it's not ideal for family time, but sometimes the only sensible course of action is to parent in shifts – one parent has your baby, the other has a rest. It was when George was two weeks old that my husband and I first cottoned on to this – until that point we had both got up for him in the night, and consequently we were both exhausted. My husband headed off to the guest room for an eight-hour catch up, and the following night I did the same. I remember feeling high on sleep after my night off – I was so much more myself.

Obviously, night-time arrangements depend on your circumstances; for example, if one parent is working and the other isn't, the working parent often doesn't get up in the night. You need to find a system that works for you, one that allows both parents to get some decent rest. However, do make sure there's some sense of fairness – if Dad works all week, he can still help out at the weekends, for example.

'Marie and I split each night into two. She's always gone to bed earlier than me, so it made sense for her to head to bed around eight or nine, after Michael's bedtime feed, and then I would be "on duty" until midnight and give him late evening feed. Then I got seven hours sleep, and Marie got up in the night. Usually, Michael wouldn't wake until three or four, so Marie got a decent six to seven hours sleep as well. Okay, it meant we gave up watching tele together till late, but it was worth it because we could manage the tiredness.'
Blake, dad to Michael

In the day, consider finding ways to give both parents some time off. It's not always possible on a week day if one or both parents are working, but certainly at weekends you could take it in turns to have a lie in. It's not selfish; sleep is essential.

Relaxing to re-energise
Sleep may not be possible, but is relaxation? Okay, it's not quite as restorative as a nap or eight hours in bed, but calm, quiet time with your eyes closed can really make a difference. Try to catch some time for yourself for a few minutes several times a day – while feeding your baby, while on a train or a bus, while in the bath. Even just a minute in which you close off the world and rest in your mind can press the giant 'reset' button in your body.

Also consider whether you're doing activities that are unnecessarily wearing you out. Are you trying to keep the house immaculate? Are you dashing about taking your baby to every baby class and group available? Are you trying to keep up with your pre-baby social life? It's easy to let looking after yourself fall down the list of priorities, but if you move it up, you find lots of areas of life easier to manage. A messy house doesn't matter. Junior won't be hindered by not attending baby boogie classes. Your friends will still invite you out in a few months if you'd rather an early night than a trip to the new salsa bar in town. All that matters is calm and relaxed parents, and thus calm and relaxed baby.

Thinking about diet and exercise
If you aren't kind to your body, it won't be kind to you. If you eat rubbish all day, or don't eat much at all; if you push yourself at the gym though you're already weary, or you sit on the sofa all day and rarely venture out – you're not helping yourself combat tiredness.

The usual advice applies: eat healthily and exercise moderately, and you'll feel energised. Plus, when you do come to climb into bed, you're more likely to sleep well.

A final note on caffeine. If you're struggling to stay awake in the day and you need to – you're going into a business meeting or driving your baby to the doctor's – a cup of coffee may be helpful. But watch your overall intake – too much caffeine and you'll struggle to sleep. As a rough guide, keep in mind that caffeine stays in the system for about six hours after consumption.

Considering quality, not quantity

So you can't get as much sleep as you'd like, but you can work on how well you sleep when you are able to crawl into bed. Consider these factors, which may be affecting your sleep:

- *Ambient noise*: Once you become a parent, you become hyper-sensitive to noise at night as you listen out for your baby. If you're not struggling to sleep because your partner's snoring or traffic outside or the hum of the boiler is irritating you, consider putting the baby monitor nearby and then putting in ear plugs. Don't panic, you'll still hear your baby (and your partner will poke you if he or she hears the baby first); but it may help you block out enough noise to sleep.
- *Anxiety*: You don't get enough sleep, and you worry about not getting enough sleep, which means you don't get enough sleep, and so on. Anxiety over lack of sleep is a common cause of insomnia. I remember putting George down and climbing back into bed, then lying awake, heart pounding, waiting for his cry. The sooner you can tell yourself to stop worrying and sleep, the sooner you'll worry less overall anyway because the anxiety is connected to exhaustion (see the earlier section 'Understanding the effects of sleep deprivation').
- *Proximity of your baby*: If your baby's in the room with you, is he too close for comfort? Babies are noisy little creatures, and if you're waking up each time he so much as sighs in his sleep, it's perhaps an idea to move the basket or crib across the room a little.

Tip: Just as you devise a wind-down routine for baby, ensure you do the same yourself. Don't expect to go from scrubbing kitchen surfaces or folding babygros to fast asleep in one fluid movement. Allow some time to yourself before bed to turn off being Mum or Dad and relax.

Reframing your ideas about sleep

I love sleep. I mean, I really love sleep. I've long loved an early night and a sleep-in, and pre-George I'd be staggering around in a fog all day if I woke just once in the night. So becoming a mummy was a bit of a shock on the sleep front. As the months went on and George didn't sleep much at night, I got pretty down about how tired I was. So because I couldn't do a great deal about getting all the sleep I wanted, I decided it was worth a try reframing my conception of lack of sleep.

It was how I felt about being tired, rather than the tiredness itself, that was getting me down. So I found positives to getting up in the night – the quietness of the house, the warm, fuzzy feeling I got that George wanted Mummy cuddles, the bliss of crawling back into bed after settling my son, knowing I could sleep now. And I realised that being tired wasn't the end of the world – it was just a feeling, and it wouldn't last forever.

> 'Sounds cheesy but I always made a point of greeting Scarlett with a big smile, especially in the mornings, regardless of what kind of night I'd had. I'm a bit sad now that she gets up by herself and doesn't wait for us to get her up. I think that providing as much love and security for the baby in their first year (and beyond) is good for them and their development.'
> Sarah, mum to Scarlet

IF ONLY SOMEONE HAD TOLD ME: ADVICE FROM PARENTS
- Babies sleep a lot. Just not when you want them to.

- Keeping a baby awake who's decided it's nap time is nigh on impossible.
- Snoring, muttering, grunting, whimpering – babies are noisy in their sleep.
- Stick a baby in a car/buggy, and he'll likely go to sleep. Which makes going out when you don't want your baby to sleep tricky.
- Tumble driers/washing machines are great pacifiers (put the baby's chair/basket on top, not inside!).
- Wake a baby before he's ready and feel his wrath!
- Don't listen to the horror stories from parents who go on and on to expectant parents that they'll never sleep or go out again. You will!

9. Batten down the hatches, baby is on the move

Rolling, sitting up, crawling, standing and walking are exciting developments, and they change the game of parenting dramatically. In the space of a few short months, you go from caring for a placid wee mite who lies quietly in your arms and stays exactly where you put her, to coping with a wriggling, wiggling, mobile baby who can get into untold mischief in the blink of an eye. It's an adjustment, but boy is it a lot of fun!

RELAXING ABOUT DEVELOPMENT MILESTONES

As I mention in Chapter 6, parents can be a competitive bunch. And, of course, we're worriers. So you can get a little preoccupied with whether baby's hitting those development milestones, and when, compared to other children.

All babies develop at different rates. Some babies are eager to explore the world – they seem to quite deliberately work out how to roll, to crawl, to walk, and are zooming about by their first birthdays. Other babies (like my George) are more chilled and watchful, and take their time. It's really not a race; and all babies get there in the end (you don't see five-year-olds crawling to school because they can't work out how to walk, now, do you?).

Tip: If your baby's in no hurry to roll or sit or crawl, don't for a moment think that it's some reflection of baby's intelligence – that your baby is, quite literally, slow. I remember one such horribly ignorant and insensitive comment directed at George when he was a baby, and I was furious. The older George gets, the more apparent it is that he's quite a thinker – so why wouldn't he have been happy to lie about and think, and take in the world around him, while a baby?

The physical development milestones for babies in the first year are as follows:

- Lift head.
- Roll over.
- Roll back over from tummy.
- Sit unaided.
- Crawl (however she likes – bum shuffle, caterpillar style on her tummy, wiggling backwards on her tummy, on all fours and so on).
- Pull up to standing, using a person or furniture for support.
- Cruise around furniture, holding on for support.
- Stand unaided.
- Walk.

Please don't take this to be a definitive list for what your baby ought to be doing by her first birthday; some babies mosey along at a leisurely pace.

There are various ways in which you can encourage baby along to the next milestone, and you can have fun with your baby in helping her take the next steps. However, I wouldn't invest too much time and energy into 'teaching' baby to develop. She'll work it out just fine on her own!

'Will didn't crawl. Or bum-shuffle. Oh no, he took a worm-like approach to travel: face down on the floor, bum up in the air, slithering along. He'd get totally filthy!' Euan, dad to William

SEEING HOW LIFE CHANGES ONCE YOUR BABY'S MOVING ABOUT

Your baby's first year is hard work simply because she changes so fast. No sooner have you got the hang of where you are in parenting than your baby changes the rules and you're back to wondering what to do. And the most rapid adjustment you make is from the day you lay your baby down on her playmat, pop into the kitchen to make a cuppa and come back to find her under the dining table or down the side of the sofa or going great guns towards the patio door.

Here's the lowdown on what to expect when it comes to your baby learning a new mode of movement:

• *Rolling over.* Such a fun one. If you happen to be watching when your baby first goes from her back to her tummy, her expression is a real Kodak moment: think Mel Gibson's face as he yells 'Freedom!' in *Braveheart*. Before long she's worked out that this rolling malarkey can get her somewhere – exciting indeed, and you have on your hands a creature who'll happily (and impressively quickly) log roll across the room.

• *Crawl.* Strictly speaking, crawl refers to hands and knees, but babies come up with their own variations on the theme. Before he crawled on hands and knees, George would shimmy across the wood floors in our house and he could get quite some distance just wiggling this way.

• *Standing and cruising.* A whole new level of your house is now within your baby's grasp – very exciting for your little one. No longer is your baby confined to finding her fun in an activity centre or play gym; now she can devise fun games for herself like crawling to the washing machine with a favourite toy and popping it in for a spin. (Tip: From now on, check the washing machine before each wash. Plastic blocks + a load of washing = expensive plumber bill.)

• *Walking.* Now the fun begins! Your baby's everywhere, and faster than you can believe. And now she's walking, she's quite happy to give climbing a try too – oh, the mischief you'll encounter!

With all of these changes, your baby goes from seeming like a very dependent creature, usually attached to Mum or Dad, to a tiny, independent person. It's a really rewarding time as a parent as you see baby's personality come through in the adventures she embarks upon.

'I remember when Kia first walked. It came from nowhere – she just took a few steps across the room to get to her rocking horse. I was so happy and proud of her. And my next thought was, "Where has my little baby gone?" She seemed so grown up all of a sudden.'
Stefan, dad to Kia

CHILDPROOFING YOUR HOME

You need to make home a safe place to be for your baby – so she's okay to explore, and so that you can leave her unattended briefly without worrying something awful's going to happen, like her falling down the stairs or fiddling with the bleach bottle under the sink. Childproofing is really just common sense – the easiest approach is to get down on your hands and knees in each room and identify the dangers that are at your baby's level (and don't forget that once she stands and climbs her reach is much higher).

Tip: Don't go over the top with childproofing. You don't need to put away every ornament in your home just in case. Your baby wants to live in a home, not an empty box! The more you watch your baby move, the more you intuitively know what needs to be out of bounds.

The main dangers you need to protect your baby from are electrocution, strangulation, suffocation, burns, falling, getting crushed and choking or swallowing something harmful. The Baby Centre website (www.babycentre.co.uk) contains a useful checklist of areas of your home to consider.

Do your best to childproof, but remember that you learn by experience. Most parents will at some point fail in childproofing and either spot the baby heading for an issue and swoop in to the rescue, or realise after the fact that the baby's got into a pickle. It's not ideal, but as long as you've successfully childproofed against the big dangers, the hope is that no great harm is done.

'Of course I knew that once Lily was rolling over I should never leave her unattended some place high up. But I had

always laid her on bed while I ran her bedtime bath, and she'd only ever rolled from her back to her tummy, then got stuck, so I thought she'd be fine. I put pillows each side of her as a barrier, just in case. I can't have been in the bathroom more than ten seconds when there was a crash and wailing. My heart just about stopped. I ran in and she was on the floor – laminate, so hard. She was fine once I gave her a hug. But I couldn't believe she'd picked that moment to roll over and over! We have a super-king size bed. She must have rolled a good three times to fall off. It's almost like she knew!'
Jenny, mum to Lily

Tip: When childproofing your kitchen, leave one cupboard at least without a childlock on it, and fill it with things you don't mind your baby playing with – plastic containers, saucepans, wooden spoons and so on. If she has one cupboard in which to play, your baby will be less interested in the others – and she won't get frustrated and bored in the kitchen while you're cooking.

'Playpen. Brilliant invention. Somewhere to put the baby when you have to step out of the room where he'll be safe and won't get into mischief. We didn't have room for a big one with bars, so we just kept the travel cot in the lounge for a while.'
Matt, dad to Katie and Tyler

LETTING YOUR BABY EXPLORE WHEN OUT AND ABOUT
You can do a pretty good job of childproofing your house, but what happens when you go out? Well, you need to strike a balance between vigilance and standing back to let your baby experience the world herself, on her own two feet (or knees, or bottom), rather than on your hip.

Where possible, don't expect your baby to stay in her buggy or on your lap. Yes, she gets grubby when crawling about on the floor in a park or a cafe, for example, but it helps her learn about her environment, it gives her a sense of independence, and anyway, that's what baby wipes are for! And your baby may walk at a snail's pace and stop to examine every blade of grass along the way to the shops, but if you can see the fun in it and make some time for her exploration, you and your baby can have some lovely bonding time together.

Finally, when you visit other people who don't have children and whose houses are not childproofed, go armed with a huge bag of toys for distraction and keep a beady eye on Junior. It's astonishing how much mischief a little one can get into if you take your eye off the ball.

IF ONLY SOMEONE HAD TOLD ME: ADVICE FROM PARENTS

- A cat flap is an intriguing little door for a baby.
- A newly-sitting-up baby is like a weeble – except as well as wobbling, she does fall down. She needs cushions aplenty all around.
- All electronic equipment – mobile, remote control, DVD player, TV – is fascinating!
- Babies learning to roll over often get stuck. And they don't like that a jot.
- Drawers in the kitchen are right at the height of a standing baby's head.
- If baby likes walking holding on to your fingers, prepare yourself for a few weeks of back ache.
- Just to mess with you, babies like to move things around. Expect a colander in the bath, a remote control in a handbag, a toilet roll down the toilet, a teething ring in a pot plant.
- Those little twangy doorstops? Best toy ever.
- Tidying the house is pointless until your baby's in bed.
- You'll likely trip over the stairgate at least once.

10. Coping with illness

Babies don't start life with hardy immune systems, so in their first year you can expect the odd bout of illness. It's heartbreaking to see baby poorly, and can be pretty wearing on Mum and Dad because baby is needier and doesn't sleep well. Usually, the baby bounces back within a few days, though, so everyone's feeling themselves again soon.

This chapter takes you through the illnesses you commonly encounter during your baby's first year, and how you can help your baby through them. I explain when to see a doctor, why scrubbing your house from top to bottom may not be the way forward (hooray), and how both you and your baby can best get through poorly periods.

FOLLOWING YOUR INSTINCTS

Before I get into discussing babies and illness in this chapter, I want to make the point that the best thing you can do for your baby when it comes to illness is to have faith in your instincts. You know your baby and you know when something isn't right. And sometimes you have to be prepared to be pushy to make sure your child gets what he needs. I learnt this when my son was seven months old and became seriously ill. It was thanks to me pestering medical staff and insisting that he wasn't right that his illness was diagnosed in time for life-saving treatment.

So if you're worried about your baby at all, see a medical professional. Don't be afraid that you'll be dismissed as a neurotic, overprotective first-time parent. It doesn't matter what people think; what matters is that you listen to your instincts. Even if it turns out that your baby's fine (and of course you hope he is), better that than worry about looking silly and risk your baby not being okay. And if you take your baby to see a doctor and you're not happy with the result, take him again, and again if necessary, and get a second opinion.

'Alex suffered from pyloric stenosis (a condition that causes severe projectile vomiting in young babies). With him being my second baby I knew after a few weeks that something wasn't right with his feeding. He would cover me, himself and surrounding areas with milky vomit which would come out at enormous force, it was horrible. I went to the doctor several times, just to be sent back with various reflux drugs. In the end, he needed some hospital treatment. So I would say if you know something isn't right then make sure you keep going back to the doctor until the problem is resolved.'

Emma, mum to Toby and Alex

ILLNESS AND YOUR BABY: KNOWING WHAT TO EXPECT

The following sections look at illnesses and ailments commonly encountered during the first year. I offer a few tips, but you can find out much more about how to help your baby on websites such as NHS Direct and Baby Centre (see the Useful Resources section at the end of the book), and of course by talking to your GP, health visitor and pharmacist.

Cold

Your baby is streaming snot (delightful). Some babies are cheery regardless; some take the 'man flu' approach and grunt and grumble. The problem with colds in babies is that they don't know how to blow their noses, so you need to find ways to help their snot drain away. Here are some ideas:

• There's a handy little device you can buy in good chemists that allow you to suck the snot out of your baby's nose (it's not as gross as it sounds – you don't suck it right to your own mouth).

• From the age of around three months (check the label on packaging), you can use a vapour rub or decongestant capsules that you sprinkle on your baby's pillow.

• Try tilting your baby slightly at night by placing a book or a towel under the head end of the mattress – then he isn't lying flat, and his nose has a chance to drain. (Note the word slightly in the previous sentence – the objective is to raise your baby's head a little, not create a night-time slide that plummets him to the bottom of his bed.)

'When Tessa has a cold I take her in the bathroom and run the shower until the room is really steamy. She's less congested then.'
Sam, mum to Tessa

Colic
Colic – prolonged, uncontrollable crying – can start at about two to four weeks and is over by three or four months old. Head over to Chapter 4 (pages 72–3) for the lowdown on colic.

Constipation
Baby's red-faced and straining while doing a poo... constipated, you think. Well, no, not necessarily. For some babies, that's simply their style. But if baby is getting distressed while trying to poo, that's a sign of constipation. Other signs include loss of appetite, a hard stomach, passing hard pellets and only doing a number two twice a week or less. The usual recommended home remedies are encouraging your baby to drink plenty of fluids, and bicycling your baby's legs to help get his digestive system moving. If you're worried, see a doctor.

Cough/wheeze
Some babies develop little coughs and/or wheezes, and these can develop into nastier problems like chest infections. With anything connected to respiration, it's best to seek medical advice.

Tip: If baby starts emitting a strange sound that's a bit like a barking seal, don't panic – he may have croup. It's pretty rare these days, and is more common in older children. Most cases of croup clear up on their own in a day or two (George had it for one day only), but it's best to see your doctor because this is an illness that affects breathing.

Ear infection

If you've ever had an ear infection, you'll know how miserable the pain is. Most ear infections are preceded by a runny nose – the cold causes the middle ear to swell up, trapping fluid, which then becomes infected. Symptoms of ear infection in babies include getting distressed while feeding (swallowing can be painful), tugging at the ear and generally being in a filthy mood. If you suspect an ear infection, take baby straight to the doctor's.

Dry skin

Babies often get patches of dry skin, especially young ones. Your health visitor or GP can recommend which creams to use – usually an emollient. Sometimes dry skin is eczema, and you need to see the doctor about the best way to treat this.

Your baby is also likely to get cradle cap at some point – dry scales/flakes on the scalp. Try to resist picking them off; use a shampoo designed for this problem or simply rub a little olive oil into your baby's scalp and the scales usually fall off the next day.

'My mother recommended adding baby oil to bath water to treat dry skin. What she didn't tell was to use only a few drops or you end up with a baby that's as slippery as an eel! It took both me and my wife to catch Steven slithering about in the bath after that treatment.'
Carl, dad to Steven, Sally and Sebastian

Eye infection

Little babies often get gunky eyes – a little yellow discharge comes from the inside corner of the eye. Sometimes this is caused by a cold; sometimes it's the sign of an infection. When you first notice the gunk, wipe it away with some cotton wool dipped in cooled, boiled water or, if you're breastfeeding, a little breast milk. If it reoccurs, take your baby to the doctor. Sticky, watery and/or pink eyes are usually a sign of an infection, such as conjunctivitis, which is super contagious – so wash your hands after any contact with your baby's eyes.

Fever
Not an illness in itself, but a symptom of an illness. If you get through your baby's first year without him ever getting a temperature, you have an exceptionally resilient child! A healthy baby has a temperature of around 36 to 37 degrees Celsius; a fever is when your baby is hotter than this. You can often tell when a baby is hot just by feeling his skin, but it's best to get a proper reading as well.

Tip: Invest in a good thermometer so you can accurately determine your baby's temperature. I worked my way through many different types, and now use an ear thermometer.

If your baby is too hot, strip him down. Encourage him to have fluids – milk and/or water. And if he's over three months of age, you can give him a dose of infant paracetamol or ibuprofen.

If you're worried about your baby – and especially if his temperature is high (38 degrees Celsius or above under three months, and 39 degrees Celsius or above for three months to one year), take him to see your doctor. Your doctor will never complain if you ask him to check a baby with a temperature.

Nappy rash
Okay, it doesn't sound like much of a problem, but nappy rash can get pretty nasty sometimes, especially if baby has diarrhoea. You can buy various creams to help with nappy rash, but the best remedy is fresh air. So if your baby's bottom is getting sore, brave a bit of nappy-free time. The worst that's going to happen is a bit of a mess (and once you hit potty training, you get used to that!).

Teething

Just when you're getting the hang of parenting and your baby's settling down, along comes teething. Some babies are born with teeth, some don't get their first tooth until they're at their first birthday – but most babies start teething at around three to six months. And the likelihood is, you and Junior won't find early teething a pleasurable experience.

If you've ever had toothache, you'll know how miserable it is. Your poor little mite can be pretty uncomfortable as teeth move down in his gums and then finally break through. The good news is, it's only usually the first year that your baby finds teething a bother – although teeth come through later, toddlers don't seem to suffer as much.

Here are some signs that your baby's teething:
- Bright red, hot cheeks.
- Desire to chew hard on things (often your finger).
- Excessive drooling.
- Irritability and distress.
- Off his food or milk (seems uncomfortable to eat).

Often, you can put a finger into baby's mouth and feel the source of the problem – a tooth pressing hard under the gum – and if you take a look you can see the white of the tooth through the thinning skin. Then one day, hallelujah, you spot/feel a tiny prick of white, and the tooth is all but through.

In the meantime, here are some ways to soothe a grumpy teething baby:
- Give him something hard to chew on – a teething ring, a flannel, a carrot (watch him for choking, though) – so he can grind down the gum and help the tooth come through.
- Soothe his aching gums with a drink of cool water, or some cold fruit puree or yoghurt.
- Once he's old enough (check packaging), try teething remedies such as homeopathic powders and numbing gels that you rub on the gums.

- If he's really struggling and he's three months old or more, he can have some infant paracetamol or ibuprofen.

'Ethan would chew on an ice lolly – I made them myself with a little apple juice mixed with water.'
Emma, mum to Ethan

Myth buster: If your baby's grumpy, he's teething. If he's off his food, he's teething. If he's hot, he's teething. Don't blame teething for every mood and ailment your baby gets. Make sure he's well in himself before putting a symptom down to teething. And try not to dose baby with painkillers every time he's grizzling – ideally, use drugs as a last resort, because doctors don't advise using over-the-counter medicines too regularly.

Upset stomach
By which I mean tummy ache or diarrhoea or sickness. Babies have delicate little digestive systems, and they can get upset easily. Make sure baby has plenty of fluids, and if he's on solids, either stick to milk feeds or to bland, easily digestible food like porridge or Weetabix. If you're breastfeeding, consider the foods you have eaten recently and whether there's a pattern to the tummy upsets – perhaps you love curry, but your baby's system doesn't.

Most upsets clear up on their own in a few hours; if your baby's lingers, ask a doctor for advice.

'At one point my wife didn't just pack spare clothes for Jo in the nappy bag – we had a change of clothes each in there too. Seems a bit extreme, perhaps... but had you been there at the Great Nappy Explosion of 2011, which took place in church service, you'd know why.'
Phillip, dad to Jo

KNOWING WHEN TO SEE A DOCTOR

You need to take your baby to see the doctor whenever you're worried – if you've a squirming feeling inside that something's not right, get him checked. And regardless of circumstance, always get your baby to the doctor if he has:

- A barking cough.
- A high fever.
- A rash.
- A swollen or sunken fontanelle (the soft bit on the top of the baby's head).
- Blood in his vomit or poo.
- Persistent vomiting and/or diarrhoea (lasting more than 12 hours).
- Pink, watery or gunky eyes.
- Strange discharge from orifices.

Also take a trip to the doctor if your baby's refused to eat or drink for more than eight hours, if he's really out of sorts or if he's crying in a way that sounds to you like he's in pain (parents know best, remember).

Finally, if you notice any of the following in your baby, don't bother with the GP, call an ambulance right away:

- Limp and unresponsive (semi-conscious or unconscious).
- Seizure activity – convulsing and/or staring vacantly.
- Struggling to breathe (look for a blue tinge to the lips).
- Meningitis symptoms: a rash that doesn't disappear when you press a glass on it, a fever (though often hands and feet are cold), rapid breathing, stiff neck, drowsy and limp, doesn't like bright lights.

Tip: If you're really worried about your baby, just call for help. Don't worry that you may be overreacting. No one will judge you for doing what you think is best for your child, and with babies, it's important to err on the side of caution.

144

PROTECTING YOUR BABY FROM ILLNESS
All parents wish their children never got ill. It's terrible to see your little one in pain or uncomfortable, and if you're anything like me, you'd rather it were you feeling poorly. So what can you do to ward off illness?

Building baby's defences
Your aim is to build up your baby's immune system. So he needs enough sleep, a healthy diet and some fresh air and daylight on a regular basis. He needs you to protect him from obvious sources of illness – so you use good food hygiene practices when preparing food (for more info, visit this website www.nhs.uk/livewell/homehygiene), you don't smoke around him, you don't take him to visit a poorly friend and so on. And your baby needs to come into contact with some germs.

Um, hang on, you're thinking, surely I want to protect my baby from germs? Well, yes – ideally your house is clean, you wipe a highchair in a cafe before your baby eats his lunch in it, you deter him from chewing on a bit of litter he's picked up off the ground. But what you don't need to be is fastidious, especially as he gets older. If you disinfect everything your baby ever comes into contact with, his little immune system has no chance to develop immunity to bugs. He needs a bit of exposure, so keep things clean, but don't get obsessed with every speck of dirt. (Keep in mind, as well, that obsessing over cleanliness may lead your child to grow up a bit inhibited and worried – he wants to explore the world and get good and messy, and to a point, you're best letting him.)

Getting vaccinations
The NHS strongly recommends that all babies have immunisations that protect against these infectious diseases: diphtheria, haemophilus influenzae type b (Hib), measles, meningitis C, mumps, whooping cough (pertussis), pneumococcus, polio, rubella and tetanus. You will be asked to take your baby for

vaccinations four times in his first year: at two months, three months, four months and between twelve and thirteen months.

Usually, the nurse at your GP practice administers the injection(s). It's not nice, as a parent, standing by while someone hurts your baby – but it's over quickly, and your baby will soon settle down afterwards with a cuddle.

The vast majority of parents permit their children to have vaccinations to prevent illnesses that are, thanks to the marvels of modern medicine, now preventable. Some parents have concerns over the side effects of vaccinations. Remember that all vaccinations have been stringently tested before use, and they greatly decrease the incidence of infectious illness. When it comes to vaccinations, you need to make an informed decision. Your GP will be happy to answer any questions you have on the subject, and to direct you to sources of information that help you understand the vaccinations.

SOOTHING YOUR BABY THROUGH ILLNESS

Poor baby. He's feeling rubbish, and there's nothing he can do about it. And you may feel pretty powerless to help your baby too. But even if you can't wave a magic wand and cure your baby, you can soothe him through his illness.

What your baby needs while he's ill is lots of attention and affection. He doesn't want to play on his own; he wants to be on your hip. He doesn't want to feed himself his lunch; he wants you to feed him. He doesn't want to sleep alone in his bed; he wants to sleep with you, in yours.

My advice for when your baby's ill is to just let go. Don't worry about the list of jobs you want to get done; just cuddle up on the sofa with your baby. And as for rules and routines, if you're making yourself and your baby miserable trying to enforce them, I say bin them for now. For example ,say you've been sleep training your baby (see Chapter 8) and now he's poorly – this really isn't the time to leave him to cry, or expect him to settle himself to sleep if he's feeling rubbish. Be lovely, cuddly, comforting, soothing Mum or Dad for now; you can put your firm-and-in-control hat back on when your baby's all better.

> 'For my first three children, I would be up and down like a yo-yo at night when they were ill. Then, for Marie, my fourth, I decided to take her into bed with me when she was really unsettled. We both slept better for it. Of course she didn't like going back in her own bed once she was better, but after a couple of nights she'd give up grumbling.'
> Lorna, mum to four grown-up children

HAVING SOME TIME OUT WHEN YOUR BABY'S POORLY

But what about you? Looking after an ill baby is no fun. My friend and I used to ring each other up when our boys were ill (which was a regular occurrence in their first winter) and all one would need to say to the other, usually in an exasperated tone, was, 'He's ill again.' We knew how each other felt when the baby was ill – exhausted and frustrated!

There seems to be a bit of a taboo on parents admitting when they're struggling. People expect, I think, that when a baby's ill, as a parent you become entirely selfless and some kind of Florence-Nightingale-esque nurse. Of course, you love your baby and you do your best to be loving and patient, but you also have your own needs and you don't feel happy when your baby's ill. Think of it this way, when your partner's got flu, how long is it before your patience wears a little thin? Of course, some people are wonderfully good at looking after poorly people, but I think a lot of us run out of steam after a while.

Unwell babies are demanding and clingy babies. What you need, as a parent, is a little time out now and again – some time to yourself to recharge. Take turns with your partner to look after the baby when you can; even if Dad comes home from work and just takes over for half an hour while Mum has a relaxing bath, it

147

makes a difference. Also don't be afraid to ask other people – friends and family – for help if you need it.

MUM/DAD'S ILL! NOW WHAT?

Nightmare! Looking after a baby is hard enough, without doing so between sprints to the toilet or through a fog of migraine.

Tip: If you feel really bad, ask for help. Soldiering on doesn't help you get well.

If you're not in a position to have someone come and help out with Junior then employ the 'by any means necessary' parenting tactic. Crawl through the day until you can put your baby to bed (and do so early!). It really doesn't matter today whether your baby's still in his pyjamas or has watched back to back Baby TV rather than doing the nice craft activities you had planned – choose the easiest path and look after yourself as best you can.

And if baby AND Mum AND Dad are poorly, well then you're really in a pickle. Send an SOS to friends and family; and if that fails, I suggest a tag team approach, so both parents get some opportunity to rest. Remember, it won't last long!

IF ONLY SOMEONE HAD TOLD ME: ADVICE FROM PARENTS

• Always been repulsed by babies with crusty, snotty noses? Prepare to have your very own now. And the more you wipe it, the more it flows – and the more cross Junior gets at you wiping.

• A teething baby chomping on your finger has an impressive bite.

• Put on a nice, clean, white, expensive shirt and your baby sees that as a signal to throw up on it. Copiously.

• Give a sicky baby a milk feed too soon after he vomits and back up it comes, sometimes with projectile force.

• In the first year as a parent, you may get ill a whole lot more. What your baby catches, you often catch too. Joy.

• Poorly babies sleep a lot. Just not necessarily when you want them to.

• There are no limits when it comes to where diarrhoea will spread. Armpits. Between toes. Hair.

• When doctors and health visitors ask 'Is this your first?' the subtext may be 'If so, you're incompetent/ignorant/paranoid'. If you get that vibe, stand tall. You know your baby!

11. Having a life of your own

This is a short chapter, but an important one. Because it's all about making yourself happy. And if parent's happy, baby's happy.

Babies are lovely, but especially for the principal caregiver, they do rather take over your life and you can end up losing track of who you are beyond being a parent. This chapter focuses on helping you keep/rediscover a sense of yourself and, crucially, doing so without guilt.

REALISING THAT YOU NEED TO BE MORE THAN MUM/DAD

Being a parent is wonderful – rewarding, amusing, fulfilling, a privilege. No doubt you'll agree that some of the best moments in your life are moments with your child – when she smiles at you, when you hold her close for a sleepy cuddle, when you catch her posting a jam sandwich into the video recorder and she gives you that mischievous grin.

But as much as you love your child, being a parent isn't all you are, and it isn't all you want from your life. And that's okay.

Yes, your baby needs you to be an attentive and loving parent. But she also needs to grow up to see that you are a separate person, not simply put on this planet to meet her needs. By being yourself, and having interests and passions outside of parenting, you free your child to grow up to do the same – you empower and inspire her.

For example, think of the following aspects of your life outside of parenting, and how by pursuing these elements of your life you are a good role model who inspires and informs your child's development:

- *Culture* (e.g. parent enjoys films/art/theatre/music): Develops an interest in the world around and in forms of expression; encourages creativity.

- *Social* (e.g. parent socialises with friends and family): Develops social skills, essential to getting on in all aspects of adult life.
- *Sport* (e.g. parent plays or watches tennis or football or rugby): Develops sense of team work and discipline.
- *Work* (e.g. parent has a job): Develops work ethic, commitment, responsibility, tenacity, organisational skills, sense of ambition.

Clearly, much of this learning comes into play as the child gets older, but there's no reason why you can't start as you mean to go on.

'Before we even got pregnant my husband and I had an honest conversation about what life might be like after we had a baby. We both agreed that we would still want some sort of social life and agreed to support each other in that. I still go to my annual music festival whilst he's then left in charge of childcare. He has never made me feel guilty about going and I doubt he ever would. Likewise he still has the odd weekend away with his friends. Seeing our friends and having a bit of free time helps us stay sane. It's best to bear in mind, though, that you're never really off duty. Even if I'm not with my daughter and husband they're always on my mind. There is no "off" button but it's fine. I wouldn't have it any other way.'
Sarah, mum to Scarlet

'It's important to me that my son grows up to see that his parents work hard for the family, and that we're interested in lots of things in the world. I want him to become a hard-working, energetic adult who's really engaged with people. And the best way to achieve that is for me and his mum to model the behaviour.'
Clarke, dad to Lawrence

LETTING GO OF GUILT

You spend a morning with a client rather than playing with your baby. How do you feel? Guilty. You go out with your partner and leave your baby with a babysitter. How do you feel? Guilty. You read a book for half an hour while your baby kicks about alone under her play gym. How do you feel? Guilty.

Guilt seems to be intrinsic for many parents. You feel, somehow, like space for you isn't allowed – that giving some of your time and energy to something that pleases you is selfish.

But a degree of separation is necessary as your baby grows up. When your baby's a few hours old you probably feel like you don't want anyone to hold her for long – you're very protective, and you're tied together tightly. That's natural, of course. But as your baby grows up, your job as a parent is to let her, slowly and gently, become an independent person – and making her the sole focus of your life and spending all of your time with her doesn't help her develop a sense of herself, or the skills she needs to cope in the world as she gets older.

You're the parent: you make the rules. It's all about balance – striking the happy medium between being with your baby and having some space for yourself. Of course, the baby gets the lion's share of your time; but even an hour or two a week spent on what interests you can really help you feel happier as a parent.

Tip: Having a life of your own and parenting don't need to be mutually exclusive. Love long walks in the country? Buy a baby carrier, pop her in and off you go. Want to see a film? Head to a parent and baby screening. Invited to a friend's thirtieth? Bring your baby. What you take your baby along to depends on the circumstances, but being a parent doesn't need to mean spending all of your days at home, at a baby group or at a playground – your baby enjoys seeing the big wide world as well.

'The first time Steve and I went out and left Becky with my mum to babysit, I was a basket case! I mean, it was my mum looking after her, so I had nothing to worry about, but it felt so wrong to be away from her. But Steve and I

hadn't had any time together for weeks, and after I'd rung Mum a few times and she kept telling me Becky was fine, I relaxed, and it did us good. Now we go out every fortnight.'
Diane, mum to Becky

THINKING BACK TO THE YEARS BB (BEFORE BABY)

I don't know about you, but I spent a good deal of the first few weeks of being a parent reminiscing about life BB – when I could sleep all night, when I could eat a meal in a leisurely fashion, when I could stay awake through an entire episode of *CSI* and follow the plot! Some days, I wondered if I'd ever live like that again. The good news is, the answer was yes!

When thinking about how you can keep a sense of yourself as a parent, consider the things you miss from BB – which of these you can happily give up now (perhaps lengthy drinking sessions on a Friday night, and the subsequent Saturday hangover), and which you'd like to keep in your life. For example, you may decide you still want to go to the gym, or watch footie with your mates now and again, or see the latest films at the cinema, or meet with friends regularly. You may not be able to fit as many activities in as you used to, but there's no reason why you shouldn't build in some of your hobbies and passions – and add to them as your baby gets older and less needy.

'I've been playing football every Monday evening since my teens. After Jake was born I took a break so I was home to help out, but after a few weeks I realised I really missed it. It's only an hour and a half once a week, but I think it keeps me sane!'
Martin, dad to Jake

THE SKY'S THE LIMIT

Becoming a parent is a transformative experience – you learn a lot about yourself, and you may even find you change a little; for example, you're more loving, or more relaxed, or less interested in working. And you can build on this development, if you want.

For example, as well as being a mum, I wear two other hats: I'm a writer, and I'm a businesswoman. It took me some time after I had George to realise it was okay to keep pursuing these paths in my life – that I wasn't being selfish or a bad mum. Many friends who are also creative and self-employed, and who don't have children yet, tell me that they worry becoming a parent will knock them off course – that their businesses will fold; that they'll struggle to be innovative and creative. I'm not denying that it's more of a challenge when you're tired, and you have to learn to manage your time better so that your baby gets plenty of attention and time, as well as your other pursuits. But having a baby needn't hold you back from anything you want to achieve.

And as well as your existing aspirations, you may find new areas you want to explore. Just being a parent can lead you to new interests; for example, baking, crafts, helping at a baby group, growing veggies, visiting museums.

Whatever you do, make it a positive aspect to your parenting, not a guilty pleasure.

'First babies are totally portable – to parties, pubs, the cinema, restaurants, and on holidays. When Kitty was little we used to take her everywhere with us, to pubs, parties and restaurants, so in a sense our social life didn't alter that much. Make the most of trips out during the day (and evening) with your first one – Kitty and I used to go out exploring, visiting museums, friends, Legoland, farms and all sorts, sometimes leaving in the early morning and coming home at night after meeting my husband or friends for dinner, but by the time Ted came along Kitty was at school so we were tied to school times.'
Nicci, mum to Kitty, Ted and Florence

IF ONLY SOMEONE HAD TOLD ME: ADVICE FROM PARENTS

- If you're going out with friends, take a break from parenting. It's easy to spend the whole evening talking baby, baby, baby!
- Baby ear protectors: ideal for festivals and loud events.
- Take a baby out somewhere lively and she'll love the buzz and the sights. Keep her out hour after hour and she'll flick a switch from fascinated to overstimulated and narky faster than you can say, 'Look, poppet, another firework.'
- You've a right to go out and about with your baby. Perfect your 'And your problem is?' haughty look to fire at the 'never-had-kids-and-don't-like-the-noise-they-make' people you come across.

12. Handling work and childcare, or the lack of either

Life for 1950s parents was very different. Dad went out to work; Mum stayed at home with the children. Simples. But where was the choice?

So along came the women's liberation movement of the 1960s to 1980s, and it transformed family life. Now, women could choose to work – and they did, in their masses. Fast forward to the 2010s and we have a situation where both women and men work. There's a down side to this change: many mums and dads actually have little choice about working, because to do otherwise would lead to financial hardship. But on the plus side, we now live in a more equal society where Mum can work if she wants to and Dad can take a more active role in bringing up the children.

In this chapter, I look at going out to work versus staying at home, and having someone else look after your baby. These are tough aspects of parenting, and they have a big emotional impact. Hopefully, by the end of this chapter you've found some peace in the decisions you make.

BEING A WORKING PARENT

Of course, any parent is a working parent – parenting is hard work! But in this section, I'm referring to being a parent who has a job. Once maternity/paternity leave is over, you need to work out how things are going to be – who's going to work, and when?

Deciding who's going to work

You have several options. Here are the main ones:
- One parent stays home with your baby full time, while the other works full time.

- One parent works part time and has your baby the rest of the week, while the other works full time.
- Both parents work full time.
- Both parents work part time at different times.

Your decision depends on these factors:

- *Career progression*: Perhaps one of you is climbing the career ladder, and can't afford to take months or years off to stay at home.
- *Job set-up*: It very much depends on what jobs you have. Who's the higher earner? Who's got the more flexible job? Who's got the most secure job? Can either of you go part time?
- *Money*: How much income do you need to meet your outgoings? What can you afford in terms of time off to care for the baby? Is it worth working given the cost of childcare? You may decide to tighten your belt so that one parent can work less or not at all, or you may find that you both need to work.
- *Personal fulfilment*: As a parent you may want to work – because you enjoy it, because you're ambitious, because it's not your idea of fun hanging about the house with your baby all day.
- *Views on your baby's care*: You may have strong opinions on how you want your baby to grow up – you may really want your baby to go to nursery, so she learns to socialise with others; or you may feel strongly that you want time with your baby during the week.

Tip: Remember that many employers subscribe to the childcare vouchers scheme, which allows you to save around £1,000 per year in tax. Check out www.childcarevouchers.co.uk and www.hmrc.gov.uk/childcare for more information.

Re-jigging your working week
Working needn't mean nine-to-five, Monday to Friday. You may be able to rearrange your hours to allow more time with your baby.

Under UK law, mums and dads can apply to their employer for flexible working as long as they've been in their employment for 26 weeks. Flexible working can mean:
- Flexi-time – working a total number of hours spread over a core period and then your choice of hours.
- Going part time.
- Job sharing – often with another parent.
- Squeezing your working week into fewer days, for example Monday to Thursday.
- Working from home one or more days a week.

You have to put together a strong case for your employer to show both why you need flexible working and how it won't be detrimental to the business. Your employer can only reject your application if there is a good business reason to do so.

'My wife Michelle was finding it hard work at home with our twin boys. I was nervous about asking my boss whether I could work at home one day a week, but I decided nothing ventured... He was actually really good about it, and now I work at home on a Wednesday to break up the week for her. It's not a skive day – I do actually work! But I get to help out more, and have meals with them all. And I finish work at half four and take over.'
Martin, dad to Blake and Nathan

If you're self-employed rather than employed, of course, flexible working is a whole lot easier. You can come up with a new working routine that allows you more time with your baby.

Dealing with your feelings

Guilt is a big problem for many parents who work – you feel bad because you're working instead of looking after your baby; you worry that you've prioritised career or money over your baby's wellbeing; you feel it's wrong somehow if you know, deep down, that you need to work in order to feel happy and fulfilled, and to have a break from parenting.

If this sounds familiar, take a look at Chapter 11, which is about having a life of your own outside of being a parent. As long as you're spending some time with your baby, and showering him with love, you're not doing anything wrong by working. Your baby needs to grow up to see that people work for a living, to see that we take responsibility for ourselves and provide for our families.

LOOKING AT CHILDCARE OPTIONS

If both parents are going to be at work for periods in the week – whether all day, every day, or just a morning or two – you need some childcare support. The following sections help you think through what'll work for your family.

Knowing what kinds of childcare are available

Most parents prefer to look after baby themselves until he's three months of age; indeed, many caregivers won't take younger babies. Between the age of three months and one year, you may decide to get some childcare for baby – either because you need to work, or for a little time out. You have four options:

- *Childminder.* Your baby is looked after at the childminder's home, usually alongside other children (sometimes including the childminder's own). A childminder is only allowed to look after three children under the age of five.
- *Friend/family member.* Care may be in your home or your friend/family member's home. Note: if you leave your baby at a friend's house for more than two hours a

day and you pay that friend for the childcare, by law the friend has to be Ofsted registered as a childcare provider.
• *Nanny*: Comes to your home to look after your baby, and depending on your preference, may also take him to baby groups and out on play dates.
• *Nursery*: Can be in workplaces, or privately run. Look after children from baby to age five.

Here are some aspects to consider when comparing your options:
• Trained in child development and first aid? All may be; nursery staff certainly are. But friends and family are unlikely to be.
• Inspected by Ofsted? Yes for childminders and nurseries; no for nannies and friends/family.
• Criminal Records Bureau check? Yes for childminders and nurseries; no for nannies and friends/family.
• Safety of premises ensured? Yes for all, expect perhaps friends and family.
• Costs less than £5 per hour? This is usually the case for a childminder and nursery (but not always); nannies cost more.
• Payment? All should accept payment by cash, cheque or bank transfer. A friend or family member may offer free childcare. A nursery and a childminder may accept childcare vouchers. A nanny is a bit trickier. If the nanny works for more than one family, she's self-employed and pays her own tax. If she works only for your family then you're her employer, and you pay her a salary and take care of her tax. For more information, check out the website www.nannytax.co.uk.
• Home environment? All except the nursery offer childcare in a home environment.
• Interaction with other children? Possible with all options (the childminder may have other children to look after; the friend or family member may have their own

children; the nanny may be happy to take the baby to baby groups), but certainly on a larger scale at a nursery.

• Available every day, regardless of illness? Only a nursery is unaffected by illness – a nanny, a childminder and a friend or family member may have to pull out of looking after your baby due to illness.

• Will look after your baby when he's ill? Childminders and nurseries won't; nannies and friends and family may do.

• Available for out-of-hours babysitting? Friends and family, childminders and nannies may offer this option; a nursery is unlikely to, although you may find that a member of staff offers this service independently of the nursery.

Tip: To find out what childcare options are available in your area, do a web search and contact the Family Information Service (FIS) – the website www.daycaretrust.org.uk has a handy tool for finding your local FIS branch.

Choosing the best solution for you and your baby
Childcare is a very personal choice. The best way to work out what fits best for you and for baby is to explore the options that appeal to you (and remember, of course, that you can mix them up if you want; for example, a nursery in the morning and a nanny in the afternoon). That may mean visiting nurseries and childminders' homes, interviewing nannies and grilling your friend/relative over their approach to childcare.

So, what are you looking for? Well, there are the practical considerations of course – distance to home, opening hours, cost, availability, ratio of children to adults, facilities, activities on offer, quality of meals, experience and so on. In addition, here are some questions to ask yourself for each kind of childcare which help you get in touch with your instincts about a person/place:

• Is the caregiver(s) attentive and affectionate?
• How does the caregiver respond to your baby?

- How does your baby respond to the caregiver?
- Do the other children seem happy?
- Is the caregiver happy to accommodate your wishes; for example sticking to baby's routine or feeding him expressed milk?
- Is the environment clean and homely and fun?
- Is there plenty for baby to do?
- Are there structured activities?
- Can you see evidence of creativity; for example, paint handprints on the wall?
- Will the caregiver report to you after each visit what your baby's been doing?
- Can you imagine your baby having a fun day with this caregiver and in this environment?

'What made me choose our nursery? I think it was when they showed me in the baby room and all the babies were sitting around a bowl of cake mix taking turns to stir it, and they were covered in cocoa powder and they all looked like they were having a whale of time. Something about them letting the babies get a bit messy and explore told me Hina would love it there, and she does – they clean her up before she comes home, but I love to see a bit of paint or glitter on her!'
Zahra, mum to Hina

Tip: I've been on childcare from both sides of the fence – as a mum and as a childcare provider – and I know that the most important thing is to get to know the person you're considering as a caregiver. Spend some time with the potential caregiver, and give yourself a chance to determine how you feel about the person who may be looking after baby.

Making a final decision on what childcare you'll use for baby isn't easy, but your best bet is to trust your instincts. And remember that whatever you decide to do isn't set in stone. So if you try an option and it doesn't suit, you can move on and try something else. Okay, you want stability for baby, but sometimes it's not possible to make a decision about your baby's childcare at three months and stick with that set-up until school.

The key to being happy with childcare is willingness to be flexible and to listen closely to your instincts.

Dealing with your feelings

Hopefully, you've done a couple of settling-in sessions with your caregiver to ease in gently to leaving your baby for several hours. But still, day one isn't going to be easy for you, I'm afraid. Expect tears.

With a bit of luck you'll pass your baby to the caregiver and he'll be totally unphased by the transfer. But by the time you reach the car you'll likely be feeling a bit emotional. I remember sobbing the first time I drove away from George's nursery – like every metre I drove was a wrench, too far from my little boy. I felt guilty for leaving him; I felt anxious that I wouldn't know everything he was doing; I felt irrationally jealous of the Other Woman who'd be cuddling him at nap time.

The good news is, it gets easier! You become used to the new routine, and each day that you see your baby is fine and happy when you pick him up, you feel better. Soon, you'll drop him off and feel a little pang as you go, but you'll have accepted the situation. And you get to spend all day looking forward to collecting your baby, and seeing his little face light up with joy when he sees you.

Sometimes, babies are the ones who are clingy – and especially if you put your baby in nursery later rather than earlier, or during a separation anxiety phase (natural development phases during which babies become anxious about being separate from Mum and/or Dad). It's not nice stepping out of a door leaving your baby howling in outrage at your abandonment. You feel like a lousy parent. You're not. Baby'll get over it fast, with soothing and distraction from his caregiver. And often if you get the chance to peek through the window and see your baby a minute or two after you've left, you see him rolling about the floor in glee without a care in the world!

Tip: Now and again, pick up your baby early and catch the caregiver unawares – the best way to see how your baby's doing when you're not there.

STAYING AT HOME WITH YOUR BABY

Being a stay-at-home-parent has a bad rep. People think it's a cushdy life to spend your days hanging out with a tiny person. Well, yes, of course, it's lovely in many ways, and it's nice not to have to get up, put on a uniform/suit, commute to work and do as your boss says. But is it easier than going out to work? No siree. Boredom, frustration and exhaustion are often on the cards when you stay home with your baby, whether every day or part of the week.

Getting through the long days with your baby

A day alone with a baby seems to elongate – each hour ticking by slowly (unless your baby's asleep, in which case the clock seems to go into turbo speed). Spending time with your baby is of course fun, but after a long day you can find time with him a little wearing.

When the days are stretching out in front of you and you're feeling gloomy, you need to come up with a strategy that allows you to look after baby and enjoy your days. Here are some tips for stay-at-home parents:

• Get out of the house every day, even if it's just to the local park. Home can become claustrophobic after a while, and it helps to be around other people.

• Befriend other stay-at-home parents (see Chapter 6 on meeting other new parents).

• Have some kind of structure/routine to your day.

• Make sure you get time to yourself in the day (while your baby's napping) and once your partner's home (see Chapter 11 on having a life of your own).

- Think about projects you can get stuck into with your baby. Boredom is a big factor in dissatisfaction. Decorate a room, plant a vegetable garden, get into baking – anything hands-on you can do in the day while your baby's with you.

'Sometimes days at home alone with a baby can feel very lonely and isolating. The best tip I can give is to get out of the house as much as possible. I used to drive to Bluewater just for some baby wipes rather than popping to the local shop just to get out for a whole morning!'
Maria, mum to Oliver and Thomas

Dealing with your feelings

Don't feel guilty if you sometimes struggle with being a stay-at-home parent (and equally, don't be smug if you find it a breeze!). There's nothing wrong with admitting that you don't hugely enjoy a day filled with poo and dribble and crying and baby puree thrown at you. And it's okay to admit that sometimes babies – lovely as they are – are just a little boring, and that you miss some intelligent, adult company. You're not alone; you're just a normal parent.

'I stay at home with my two boys, Alexander and Joseph. Sometimes I feel like people look down on me for this, and I find myself getting defensive and saying "I used to be a solicitor, you know" – like being a mum isn't enough. The way I cope with the day is to have plenty of activities planned, and I meet up with other mums a lot. Alex and Joe like being busy and being around other children, and I get to have a natter over a coffee, so it works for all of us. Some days I'd give anything to swap places with my partner and be the one who works, but then I know he misses out on a lot – and this time before they start school is precious.'
Beatrice, mum to Alex and Joe

'My partner had the better job, and was going places in his career, so we decided I'd be the one to do most of the childcare. I like it – for me, a day of finger painting and Pingu beats putting on a suit and sitting in an office any day. Some people seem to think I'm bonkers though. A man? At home? With a baby? Then there's the gay thing, of course. I get the odd comment that Dylan should be in daycare, around women. As far as I'm concerned, if he's with someone who loves him and plays with him, he's happy!'
Ben, dad to Dylan

IF ONLY SOMEONE HAD TOLD ME: ADVICE FROM PARENTS

• Don't bother competing with your partner over who's got it tougher – the one who works more, or the one who has the baby more. Neither of you will win.

• Nannies these days don't fly with umbrellas or tidy toys away with a click of the fingers. Shame.

• Getting your baby to nursery or the childminder's on time is an art to perfect. You get yourself ready. You get your baby ready. You get your baby's stuff for nursery ready. You de-ice the car. You get your baby strapped into the car seat. He promptly vomits all over you, him and the car, or has an exploding nappy moment.

• You need two different hats for parenting and working. Don't muddle the two and think your baby should run to schedule and work colleagues need their noses wiped.

• Remember scoffing at people who watch naff daytime TV shows – 1970s detective shows, melodramatic soaps, Jerry Springer-style chat shows? Beware; they can become strangely addictive when at home with your baby in the week.

• An hour alone with your baby can go very slowly. An hour to yourself? Gone in a flash.

- It's all too easy when faced the question, 'And what do you do?' to mutter dejectedly, 'Oh, I'm just a stay-at-home mum/dad.' Take out the just and answer with pride.

13. Focusing on your relationship

Babies put a big strain on a relationship. Couple time is often last on the list when you have a young baby, and it's all too easy to take difficult feelings out on a partner and to feel somewhat usurped in his/her affections by your bundle of joy. This chapter focuses on keeping the relationship healthy, covering compromise, communication, time together and intimacy. (If your relationship is in difficulties, or you're a single parent, take a look at Chapter 14.)

> 'As hard as it might be with a new baby, remember time for you and your partner, even an hour just the two of you, and remember I love yous! It's always lovely to hear. Don't fight against each other and try to think you're on the same team.'
> Suzanne, mum to Jay, Kyle and Vinnie

FINDING MIDDLE GROUND ON PARENTING
Hopefully, you think that you and your partner are pretty compatible, or you wouldn't be together. But just because you like the same kinds of music or both enjoy Italian food or have similar life plans doesn't mean you always agree on the best way to parent.

Disagreements can start during pregnancy (Do you find out the sex or not? Do you have an amniocentesis if the doctor suggests it? Do you paint the nursery pink, blue or yellow?). But it's usually once the baby arrives that differences in views and styles become apparent.

Here are some areas in which you and your partner may not see eye to eye:

- Caregiver: A common source of disagreement – who exactly looks after baby at a given time?
- Discipline: One partner may already be trying to shape baby's behaviour and teach wrong and right; the other may think it's far too early for all that.
- Feeding: Breast versus bottle can cause disputes, as can weaning – what your baby eats, and when.
- Play: Dad may have firm views on what your baby should play with, and that she should have structured play time; Mum may be more go-with-the-flow – or vice versa.
- Routines: One of you may like control and to organise the baby's day, while the other is quite happy floating through chaos.
- Separation: Some parents have the baby constantly in their arms/on their shoulder/on their hip; some think the baby needs some space sometimes.
- Sleep: Dad may think the baby's sleeping just fine; Mum may think the baby needs some sleep training – or vice versa.

I could go on, but you get the idea. Each parent has a unique parenting style (see Chapter 1 for more on this), and your mission is to gel together.

Parenting together is a learning curve, and in time you settle into it. The thing to remember is that in plenty of areas you need to reach a compromise; but there's also room for each parent to have a different approach. For example, you choose toys together for your baby, but you have different ways of playing with her. So Mum may like creative and messy play activities, and reading books, while Dad likes doing puzzles and building towers and giving space rocket rides in the air.

Tip: Once you iron out the areas of baby's life that you feel you must reach agreement on, try to step back and let your partner do his/her thing, even if sometimes you want to interfere. This is especially important for the parent who looks after baby most – it's easy to be critical of the way your partner cares for baby when you've got it down to a fine art. Sometimes, you just have to stand back and watch your partner wrestle with the buggy straps, rather than criticise or push him/her out of the way and take over.

> 'I think you can compromise on most things, but I also think that sometimes one parent has to defer to the other. For example I always went to Izzy at night when she cried, but eventually my husband got fed up and said we should leave her. I just couldn't – it was the strongest feeling as a mum. My husband saw how upset I got and realised this was really important to me, so he gave in. I think you just can't compromise if it goes against a strong instinct.'
> Yolanda, mum to Izzy

COMMUNICATING

Feeling low? Can't remember the last time your partner looked you right in the eye and said, 'How are you?' Frustrated that it always seems to be you getting up in the night? Wishing your partner would stop leaving the buggy in the hallway and forgetting to buy milk and winding the baby up before sleep time and sleeping through her cries?

You have a choice of three ways to deal with the situation:
1.   Say nothing. Either suffer in silence, or send passive-aggressive signals (huffing, rolling your eyes, tutting, slamming about, doing things with bad grace) to your partner in the hope he/she fathoms what's wrong.
2.   Have a row. Shout, scream, throw things. Cast hurtful accusations. Say things you don't mean.
3.   Tell your partner, in a calm and adult fashion, how you feel.

Options 1 and 2 are confusing and frustrating and pretty childish, but when you plump for Option 3 you have a better chance of having your feelings heard, and getting the response you want from your partner – and, of course, also finding out what your partner wants.

Tip: Most parents of a young baby find they snap at each other more and row more, and that's normal – you're both tired and overwrought, and you're both struggling to get your own needs met. Forgive each other if you lose your cool, but do your best to diffuse the tension and talk about what the underlying issue is, and soon you'll feel much better.

And if you can, avoid pressure mounting. Often, a simple 'How are you?' and an attentive ear makes all the difference.

Remember, a baby who sees his parents considering each other's feelings and being affectionate with each other learns that this is how relationships work, and can grow up to do the same.

'Robert and I got in this nasty cycle of rowing after Harry was born, and I began to feel like it was all falling apart. We were sniping over every little thing. We went to see a relationship counsellor, who told us we weren't talking enough (though we were shouting plenty!). It took a while to open up again. It felt a bit like I didn't trust him because I'd felt lonely for a while. We started out writing notes to each other about how we felt, then we talked. By our summer holiday [when Harry was 7 months] we weren't rowing and I wasn't worried about us anymore. In fact, I fell pregnant!'
Caitlin, mum to Harry and Bonnie

Tip: If you're feeling frustrated with your partner, watch him/her with your baby. Even if you feel your partner isn't meeting your needs right now, you hopefully see him/her being loving with your baby, and sometimes that's enough to help you feel affection, rather than irritation, once more.

MAKING TIME FOR EACH OTHER

Time is a scarce commodity when you have a baby. In fact, it's quite easy to get to bedtime and feel like you haven't had a single moment to yourself – the day is just a blur of babydom.

But time for Mum and Dad is essential – you need time together to share your feelings and thoughts, and to cement the foundation of your family: your relationship. You need to remember why you love each other, and that your being together is the whole reason the baby exists.

Of course, couple time vies with time to yourself. Sometimes, after having a baby attached to you all day, you really just want an hour to yourself in the evening, and that's fine. But also try to spend a little time together each day – even ten minutes helps. It's the quality of the time that counts – a few minutes having a cuddle and sharing feelings helps you more than an hour sitting side by side in silence staring at the TV.

Tip: Make a date night once a week. Get a babysitter, or stay home – but make sure you focus on each other, and try not to talk about your baby all night!

'Four words: babysitting circle; sanity saver.'
Mike, dad to Kate and Bryan

BEING INTIMATE

In Chapter 2, I talk about sex during pregnancy, and point out that everyone is different – some are randy; some are right off sex. This rolls right on into baby's first year. Once Mum's recovered from birth, you may soon resume your usual sexual relationship; or you may find that things are a little different now Junior's here, and either way, that's fine and normal.

All sorts of things can lessen your libido once you're a parent – exhaustion, emotions, feeling a little unsettled by the baby's presence in the house, perhaps avoiding sex because you don't want another baby right now.

In time, you feel more like yourself, and you adjust to having your baby around. But if you feel unhappy that you and your partner aren't as intimate as you'd like, perhaps you need to consider working at it a little. Before baby, sex can be spontaneous and easy; after baby, you may have to make a little effort to clear the time and space, and get into the mood.

> 'Overnight babysitting is better than evening-only if you want some alone-time with your other half. If you can get Granny to have the baby for the night, you've a better chance of really relaxing.'
> John, dad to Kayla

IF ONLY SOMEONE HAD TOLD ME: ADVICE FROM PARENTS

- Babies are sensitive and don't like seeing their parents row. Tone it down or take it outside unless you want to add a howling baby to an already stressful situation.
- 'Did you buy wipes?' 'How much milk did she take?' 'Is she having a bath tonight?' It's easy to get lost in all the practical stuff of parenting. Make some time too to enjoy your baby, and each other.
- Poo and vomit and wee and gunk become comfortable conversational topics. Watch you don't forget whose company you're in and start chatting about your baby's latest exploits in front of elderly Mr Jones from next door, or your partner's mess-phobic mother, or the vicar after Sunday service.
- Having your baby in bed with you at night is a passion killer. Having your baby in a Moses basket beside you at night is a passion killer. Having your baby in a cot in the next room and hearing every whimper and sigh on the baby monitor at night is a passion killer. The solution: find other times of day, and rooms of the house, for intimacy.

14. Coping when life doesn't go as planned

All you want is a healthy, happy family, but in some circumstances achieving this isn't easy. This chapter takes a look at difficulties that some parents encounter beyond the typical teething pains and sleep deprivation – issues that affect physical and mental health, and that cause emotional struggles. I very much hope that none of the sections in this chapter apply to you; but if so, here you can find some reassurance.

Note: Many of the problems I discuss in this chapter can be very difficult to cope with. If you find that you're struggling, and just not feeling right in yourself, there's no shame in seeking support. Various organisations offer information and guidance (see the Useful Resources section at the end of the book), and GPs and counsellors are there to help you. Don't soldier on if you're getting nowhere; ask for a helping hand.

DEALING WITH THE LEGACY OF YOUR UPBRINGING

Parenting can stir up all kinds of feelings about your own childhood, and your parents. For example, if you've lost a parent, you can find that when you first have a baby, you grieve for that parent in new ways. Or if you've had a difficult relationship with a parent, having a baby can bring back memories and bring new realisations – perhaps showing you how you don't want to parent; perhaps creating a sense of understanding and acceptance as you realise how hard your parent's job was.

If your childhood wasn't entirely happy and secure, and you find you experience difficult feelings once you're a parent, you're not alone – many parents encounter this on some level. The feelings are an opportunity to learn from the past, and to let go and move on.

There were many reasons that I wanted to have a baby, but I'd always known that in some way it would help me feel closer to my own mother, whom I lost when I was a baby. The reality was quite a shock, and in the first few months I missed my mum a great deal. I felt like I had no idea how to mother, because I had barely been mothered myself. I wished she were alive to tell me what to do; and to be there for me as I struggled. I wished George was going to have a grandmother. But in time, as I worked through the feelings, the sadness reduced, and while I'll miss my mother every day for the rest of my life, it doesn't ache as it used to.

'I had a pretty rubbish upbringing. My dad was an alcoholic, my mum left us when I was five, and I spent some of my early years in care. I so much wanted to be a dad, and to be a good one, but I was really scared that I wouldn't know how because my parents made a mess of it. My wife was excellent – she really believes in me. I also did some counselling to help me deal with my past, and to give me confidence that I wouldn't repeat the mistakes of my parents. But the best advice I can give is to just take each day – each moment, even – at a time.'
Ryan, dad to Max and Lily

COPING WITH LOSING A BABY

Losing a baby is heartbreaking. When a baby dies in the womb or at birth, nothing makes the loss okay.

I lost my second baby in the first trimester. I had what's called a silent miscarriage, which meant the baby had died but my body didn't realise this, and so as far as I was concerned, I was still pregnant. It was at 13 weeks, at my first scan, excited to see my baby wriggling about on the screen, that I was told the baby had died. It was a horrific shock, one of the worst moments of my life.

Losing a baby is just like losing anyone else in your life – it's devastating. Just because your baby wasn't born yet doesn't mean that you, as the parent, grieve it any less. You loved the baby, you dreamed of its future – to you, it was very much a part of the family. So you have to be kind to yourself, and let yourself grieve.

Something I found very frustrating after my miscarriage was to be told by well-meaning people, 'It's very common.' Yes, miscarriage happens to a lot of parents; but something in the way those words are said makes me feel there's a subtext – 'It's very common and therefore you should brush it off pretty quickly.' Loss is loss: no one has the right to tell you how you should feel when you lose a baby, and for how long you should grieve. You may feel okay in a few weeks; it may take longer. Whatever you need to go through to process the loss and let go of the baby, that's what you do.

Many parents find it helpful to have some kind of farewell to the baby. You may attend a funeral; you may have ashes to scatter – but this isn't always possible when the baby was very small. Still, you can say goodbye to baby in your own way.

'When I lost my first baby I was so upset. I was in early pregnancy, and I lost it at home, and the one thing I couldn't cope with was that there was no funeral. So my sister (who'd lost a baby too) suggested we have our own service. We went to a lake and had a memorial with songs and poems, then I lit a candle and watched it float away. Now, every year on the day the baby would have been due, I light a candle. It helps.'
Mina, mum to Alice

Support organisation: The Miscarriage Association
The Miscarriage Association offers support and information to mums and dads affected by miscarriage, ectopic pregnancy or molar pregnancy. Many people find it helpful to do or create something that marks the loss of the baby and his or her brief

life. The Miscarriage Association has the following suggestions to help with the grieving process:

- Create a certificate. Some hospitals will provide a certificate in memory of your baby if you would like this. If they don't make this offer and you would like something, ask a nurse or midwife on the ward, the hospital chaplain or the bereavement service.
- Hold a ceremony. If you didn't have a funeral or ceremony after the miscarriage, you can hold a memorial service in your place of worship, in another place that's special to you or at home. It could be just for close friends and family or even just you and your partner.
- Make an entry for your baby in your hospital's book of remembrance. The hospital chaplain will be able to arrange this.
- Plant flowers or a tree in your garden or a local garden of remembrance.
- Light a candle on anniversaries and other special days, such as International Babyloss Awareness Day, 15 October.
- Create a memory box. You could include items like your scan photo and your pregnancy journal.
- Write a letter or poem for your baby.
- Visit the Miscarriage Association website (www.miscarriageassociation.org.uk) and add message to the Forget-Me-Not Meadow or create a star on the Winter Lights of Love tree.

The big question for many parents is trying again for another baby. You may want to fall pregnant straight away or by the time the baby would have been born (some parents find comfort in the idea that the next child could not have existed had the one you lost lived); you may want to wait; you may feel you want no more children now. The choice is personal – you do what feels right for you.

HAVING A PREMATURE BABY

If baby comes a week or two early, you're all likely to be just fine. But if baby is born much too early – 32 weeks, say – then this is a very traumatic experience for parents.

You may experience all kinds of feelings:
- Angry that you're powerless to help him.
- Frustrated that you can't hold him, parent as you like or take him home.
- Not ready to be a parent.
- Robbed of the normal childbirth and early days experience.
- That you've let him down somehow.
- Worried about your baby's health.

To add to the feelings, your baby can't come home with you, and you have to live this strange half-life either in the hospital with your baby or going back and forth from home to the hospital.

This is a hugely difficult time, and you'll need to be kind to yourself as you wade through the feelings and accept support from others (check out the charity Bliss, which offers support to those affected by premature birth – see the Useful Resources section).

All that matters in the long run is that your baby is okay and comes home when he's able. Think positively, and focus on a happy ending.

> 'Anita was so tiny! She was beautiful, but not quite baby-like yet. The hardest things for us both was that we wanted to hold her, but we couldn't easily because she was in an incubator and hooked up to machines. She seemed so fragile, but over the weeks she got stronger and bigger. The day we took her home was the best day – we had a big family party to welcome her, but she slept through the whole thing. Typical!'
> Kamil and Sarah, mum to Anita

MOVING ON FROM BIRTH TRAUMA

Birth trauma is post-traumatic stress disorder caused by a traumatic childbirth experience. It can manifest as a fixation on the event (such as talking about it over and over); nightmares; flashbacks; ongoing feelings of anxiety, fear, helplessness and horror; and/or avoiding things that remind you of the event. Such symptoms make you feel pretty lousy.

Post-traumatic stress disorder is a set of normal reactions to a traumatic experience. If you have birth trauma, you aren't weak or certifiable – you're reacting normally in your mind to a bad experience you've had. Your mind is simply trying to process what happened.

I don't cover birth trauma in Chapter 3 on birth because I'm hoping you read that chapter before having your baby and are reading this one after! But if you are reading this section while pregnant, don't let it worry you – only a minority of women get birth trauma, and the best way to avoid it is to think carefully about what you need during childbirth and then make sure those around you follow your wishes – flick back to Chapter 3 for details.

If you've already had a baby then you know that childbirth is scary and difficult. Birth trauma can occur as a result of all kinds of occurrences during birth: long labour, short labour, inadequate pain relief, medical interventions, medical staff being dismissive or not listening, lack of information, lack of privacy, baby in distress, mum in distress, emergency procedures, birth of an ill or stillborn child. Aspects such as these create feelings in Mum: fear, anxiety, anger. And after birth, those feelings can linger – not only has Mum been through a physical ordeal, but she feels traumatised. In fact, she may be so distressed about her experience that she feels she can never have another baby.

The worst thing about birth trauma? Not many people realise that it exists. Mums are expected to give birth, heal physically and then cheerfully move on with their lives. So if poor Mum's still having nightmares about the birth months later, she's going to worry there's something wrong with her. There isn't!

Sometimes, all you need to move on from birth trauma is to recognise that's what you have and that it's okay and normal. But you may also find talking helpful – to your partner, to a friend or to a counsellor. Visit the Birth Trauma Association website (www.birthtraumaassociation.org.uk) for more advice.

'It was a relief, really, to be able to put a name to it. Anna just wasn't okay after the birth. She loved Alfie, of course, and was a great mum, but I could see she was struggling to put the birth experience behind her. She talked about it so often. I was there when Alfie was born, and I saw how scared and in pain Anna was, so though I didn't know how she felt, I had enormous sympathy for her. I was really proud of her for continuing to talk about it and ask for support until she felt calmer. And now we're expecting our second, I'm determined to do everything I can to help her make the next birth better.'
Jeff, dad to Alfie

COMING TO TERMS WITH ILLNESS OR DISABILITY
Every parent wants a child who's healthy. So it's devastating to discover that your baby has an illness or disability. You may experience the following feelings:

- *Anger*: Why you? Why your baby? You don't want this.
- *Anxiety for your baby*: Will he be okay? Will he survive? Will he be able to live a normal life?
- *Envy*: Others around you have healthy children; it's not fair.
- *Fear that you'll 'fail'*: You know nothing about illness/diability. Perhaps it's always made you uncomfortable. You don't know how to care for an ill/disabled child. What if you get it all wrong?
- *Helplessness*: There's no magic wand that you can wave to make it all better, and you feel it's your job as a parent to make it all better.

All these feelings are normal, and it's okay to feel them. But also be aware of the positive feelings you have about your child and about being a parent – the love.

There are lots of organisations set up to offer information, guidance and support for families affected by a particular disability or illness, and many can put you in touch with other parents in the same situation. Then you can move past the initial phase of shock and grief and fear and get to a point where you accept where you are and can see the way forward.

> 'We found out that Beth had Down's Syndrome when I was pregnant. It was an awful shock. We both struggled with our feelings – neither of us had any experience with this, and it scared us. We scared ourselves silly thinking about what life would be like. We considered termination, because we just didn't think we could cope. Then we were put in touch with the Down's Syndrome Association, which gave us loads of information, and a friend introduced us to a family she knew whose son has Down's. The more we found out, the less scared we were. I think it was the unknown that was difficult. Beth is doing great. She has the most beautiful smile.'
> Phil and Becky, parents of Beth

GETTING THROUGH POST-NATAL DEPRESSION

In the days after you have a baby, it's common to get the baby blues – feeling down and weepy and anxious. The cause: hormones, the birth experience, the shock of becoming a parent and the exhaustion. Baby blues last a few days at most, and then you feel more yourself again. But what if the depressed feelings last? Then you're in the realms of post-natal depression.

Recognising post-natal depression

Around one new mother in ten develops post-natal depression in the baby's first year. There are all sorts of reasons why you may develop this kind of depression, such as the shock of becoming a parent, altered relationships, loneliness and isolation, lack of support, hormones, birth trauma (see the earlier section on this) and childhood experiences.

Here are some of the symptoms:
- Crying often.
- Feeling down and hopeless.
- Feeling guilty about not coping.
- Feeling helpless, inadequate, unable to cope.
- Feeling hostile towards your partner and/or your baby.
- Feeling irritable.
- Feeling numb or indifferent to your husband or partner.
- Getting anxious about little things.
- Going off food, or comfort eating.
- Having panic attacks.
- Losing interest in sex.
- Obsessing over your baby's health or wellbeing.
- Struggling to sleep, waking in the night and/or having nightmares.
- Thinking about death.
- Tiredness and lethargy.
- Withdrawing from friends, family and the outside world.
- Worrying that you don't love your baby enough.

This is quite a list, and it's important to realise that you may experience just a few of these symptoms (and you're very unlikely to experience them all).

Accepting that you have post-natal depression
Even though post-natal depression is common, and it's something people know about and look for in new mothers, it's a problem that many mums struggle to admit to. It's easy to put symptoms down to tiredness. And because some of the symptoms sound really scary – like thinking about death, and perhaps thinking about harming the baby – women worry what people

will think of them if they explain how they feel. They may even be scared that the baby will be taken away from them.

If you have post-natal depression, it's important to understand that you're not going mad, and that you are very, very, very, very unlikely to harm your baby. Thoughts do not equate to actions. Also remember that there's no shame in getting post-natal depression; it's not your fault, and you're not alone – many women get it. And you won't always feel this way; with support, your depression will lift.

'Post-natal depression came as a total shock to me. I'd been fine with my first baby, Chloe – tired and emotional, of course, but still feeling that I could cope. So I expected baby number two to be the same. I quickly realised I didn't feel okay – I kept crying, I didn't want to get out of bed, I didn't even feel like cuddling Arthur much. Logically, I couldn't work out why I felt so low. Then one day Chloe said to me, "Mummy, why are you so sad all the time?" I was shocked. I thought I'd been hiding it pretty well. It made me realise that I really wasn't myself, so I told my husband (who was great) and went to see the doctor. He put me in touch with a great local support group for PND, and talking about how I felt helped – it wasn't this horrid secret any more. It took time to feel I was back to rights, but by the time Arthur took his first steps I felt like I was where I wanted to be inside and was happy again as a mum.'
Elizabeth, mum to Chloe and Arthur

Feeling better
So, what can you do to help yourself if you think you have post-natal depression? Well, first things first – be brave and go see the doctor and tell him how you feel. A diagnosis is a good starting point. Your doctor can offer treatment, ranging from counselling to medication, and you can also do things to help yourself. For example, talk to friends and family, meet up with other new

parents (see Chapter 6), get some time out from parenting (see Chapter 11 on having a life of your own and Chapter 13 on childcare options) and try to take care of yourself as best you can.

Advice for dads
It's miserable to see your partner feeling so down. You want to help, but you don't know how.

Tell her you love her, and that she'll feel better in time. Do your best to help out with your baby so she's not left alone with him too much and she can have some time off for herself. Try not to be judgmental, or take it personally if she's snappy or distant. Encourage her to see the doctor. And whatever you do, don't say the words 'Pull yourself together'. It's just not that simple for her, and she's trying her best.

> 'It was terrible seeing my wife so down after we had India. I found it hard to understand how she felt because I was so happy being a dad (tired though!). I tried to encourage her to talk about how she felt, but I think she preferred to talk to her girlfriends and her sister. So in the end I decided the best thing I could do was give her lots of help around the house and with India, so she had some space to recover.'
> Dave, dad to India

DEALING WITH RELATIONSHIP BREAKDOWN
In Chapter 12, I talk about how you can maintain your relationship while you have a young baby. But sometimes, your relationship is beyond introducing date night or communicating better, and it breaks down.

Your first concern is to be sure that there's no way to reconcile – that some time apart or some relationship counselling won't help you come back together.

But if you know that there's nothing left to save, you're faced with some difficult decisions – on both a practical and emotional level.

Often, when a relationship ends, it's every (wo)man for him(her)self. You realise you're going to be alone again, your independence kicks in and you look to ensure that you're going to be okay. This is essential, of course, but also important is how your baby will fare.

Hopefully, both Mum and Dad want to be part of the baby's life. The baby needs time with both parents, and both parents need to contribute to his upbringing. So as much as you may want to be a million miles from your ex-partner now, for your baby's sake, you need to find a way to get along sufficiently to co-parent.

Tip: Think about the relationship you want your baby to have with your ex-partner. Hopefully, while you don't love your ex now, you can see that she or he is a good parent, and you want your baby to have a good relationship with both of his parents. Focusing on ex-as-good-parent rather than ex-as-person-who-let-you-down can help diffuse tension and focus you both on the business of sharing parenting responsibilities.

So far in this section, I've touched on relationship break-downs in which both parents are to take an active role in bringing up the baby. But that's not always the case.

Your partner may have left you, and have no interest in help-ing you out with your baby. In such circumstances, it's worth having a chat with the Child Support Agency (you can get the details at www.direct.gov.uk), because your partner has a respon-sibility to provide for the child.

Alternatively, you may have no interest yourself in your ex helping out with your baby. Unless you have a good reason, if your partner wants to parent, you should let him/her – you can't cut the parent out of baby's life if he or she wants to be in it. But this does not apply when your ex is abusive. There are various organisations that offer support for people who experience domestic violence; and if you're worried for the safety of you and/or your baby, you can of course contact the police. (This advice applies to parents in abusive relationships, as well as those who have broken free.)

BEING A SINGLE PARENT

I've placed this section in the chapter on dealing with life's hiccups, because many parents don't plan to parent alone but do so because of relationship breakdown or the loss of a partner. Of course you may have chosen to be a single parent, and be quite happy as one – and that's fine.

Either way, single parenting is no picnic. It's hard work, and you can feel lonely and overwhelmed. The best approach you can have is to be willing to accepting support. Chapter 6 gives tips on how to make friends with other parents, who will understand how hard your job as parent is and can offer you support. Also reach out to support organisations and other parents in the same boat (the Useful Resources section has details of useful contacts).

When you're bringing up your baby alone, it can be hard to find confidence in your parenting abilities with no one to back you up. Hopefully, Chapter 1 in this book can help you find your feet and feel good about yourself as a parent.

And be sure to check out Chapter 11 on having a life of your own, because this is often neglected when you're single – but it's even more important to have some time out when it's just you and your baby.

> 'My husband left me while I was pregnant with our baby. It was very hard, but I understood that he still wanted to be the baby's daddy. We did our best to be grown-up about it all, though it wasn't easy. My mum was great – she stepped up and filled the gap he'd left as best she could, going with me to appointments and helping me get ready for the birth. She was there when I gave birth, and she cried – it was amazing having her there. My ex came to see Lottie in the hospital, and spent some time with her.

After that, we agreed a schedule of when he would have her and when I would have her. In the first weeks I insisted he spend time with her while I was nearby, in the house, because I felt so clingy to her, and I wasn't sure that he knew enough about babies to look after her. But he learnt, and I had to let go eventually. He still has Lottie, who's three now, every other weekend. I miss her badly when she's with him, and I worry that I'll miss out on some new thing she does, but I want her to have a relationship with her dad, and it gives me a little time to myself – time out from being a single mum, which is lonely and hard work. I'd like to think I'll have another baby one day, if I meet the right person, and that I'll have that support. But I'm lucky to have my mum helping me out, and Lottie is such a happy soul. She's worth it all.'

Jenna, mum to Lottie

Support organisation: Gingerbread

It's only natural to feel nervous about becoming a parent – especially a single parent – but with two million single mums and dads in the UK, you're not on your own. And if you ever need any practical advice or expert information, Gingerbread is here to help. Here are a few tips from Gingerbread to think about as you prepare for your new arrival:

•   Find out if you're eligible for benefits and tax credits. Call Gingerbread's Single Parent Helpline on 0808 802 0925 for expert advice.

•   Think about contact arrangements early. If you can, start talking to your child's other parent about what will work for both of you. If you need support, why not join Gingerbread's online community and chat to other single parents about their experiences?

•   Arrange child maintenance. There are different ways to set up an arrangement for child maintenance with your child's other parent and it's up to you to choose the one that best suits your circumstances. Contact Gingerbread for advice or visit www.gingerbread.org.uk.

• Don't struggle alone. Ask for help from friends and family when you need it, and call on experts for advice. Joining a local Gingerbread friendship group can be a great way to make new single parent friends and get support.

• Take time for you. Having a new baby as a single parent will be both incredibly rewarding and incredibly challenging. Don't forget to take care of yourself and build in time to eat properly, get some fresh air and take a proper break.

• Gingerbread has compiled an email advice pack for women who are pregnant and single. To receive yours straight to your inbox, visit www.gingerbread.org.uk.

IF ONLY SOMEONE HAD TOLD ME: ADVICE FROM PARENTS

• A baby's family is what you choose it to be; he doesn't necessarily need Gran, Grandad, Mum, Dad and so on – he just needs people around him who love and accept him.

• If you're struggling, you're not mad or weak – you're just a human trying to deal with experiences.

• There'll be times as a parent when you open your mouth and realise you've become your father/mother.

15. The end? Not at all! Happy first birthday

You've made it! From that first blue line on the pregnancy test to helping your little treasure blow out the candles on her first birthday cake, you're now officially no longer a 'new parent'. And your child is no longer a baby (sniff); she's a toddler now.

Once the cake is eaten and the presents unwrapped and the tired but happy little one is tucked up in bed, it's time to sit down and reflect on the last couple of years. What a journey! You remember hard times, you remember good times. Hopefully, you look back with a smile, and know that the rewards of parenting far outweigh the sacrifices you made. And now you have a sense of yourself as a parent, and have confidence in the style you've developed, based on a heap of understanding you gained along the way.

The reason that this book focuses on pregnancy to the first birthday of your first-born is that parents generally agree that this is as hard as it gets. Never again will you feel so tired, so confused, so lost. From here on, there are new challenges of course – potty training, toddler tantrums and discipline issues, for starters – but you can handle it all. And besides, there's so much fun stuff to come yet. Taking your child to see Santa; hearing 'You're the best mummy/daddy in the whole wide world'; seeing your child's little face frown in concentration as she learns to write; attempting to answer unfathomable questions like 'Why do black cats cross the road in autumn?' – so many laughs and touching moments lie ahead.

And maybe, just maybe, in time the 'Never again!' of the delivery room fades, replaced by a growing longing to do it all again. Another baby snuggled in the crook of your arm; another baby blowing raspberries because she likes to hear you laugh; another baby toddling across the room towards you, arms open wide, asking for a cuddle with a heart-melting 'Mama' or 'Dada'.

Wherever you go from here, I hope you can do so with confidence in your ability as a parent; with an understanding of what's important when bringing up a child (love, love, acceptance, and more love); and, above all, with a sense of humour.

Useful resources

No parent need be alone – there are many resources out there you can use for support and guidance. In this final section of the book, I provide details of key organisations you may turn to as a parent, and great websites to visit for information, or an online chat with other parents. And to finish off, I list some top parenting films to chill out with on a Saturday night – movies to make you smile and remind you what's great about being a mum or dad.

Don't feel you need to read this section right now (no doubt you've better things to do, like wash up a mountain of dishes or deter Junior from decorating the floor with cornflakes). But as the weeks and months go by, keep in mind that if a problem arises, there may be support for you here.

And don't forget to keep contact information for the following handy (saved on your mobile phone or stuck up on a notice board in the kitchen, for example):

- GP.
- Health visitor.
- Midwife.
- NHS Direct (England), NHS Direct Wales or NHS 24 (Scotland).
- Parenting friends you can call for support.

SUPPORT ORGANISATIONS

People recognise that being a parent can be pretty tough, so thankfully there are all sorts of organisations set up to offer support in specific areas. In this section, I provide some of the main organisations helping parents in the UK; but if you have a specific need – for example, you want to find out about child-proofing your house or you need to know all about a particular medical condition – a simple internet search will point you in the direction of plenty more resources.

Antenatal Results and Choices (ARC)
A charity offering advice and information to parents during the antenatal testing process.
Website: www.arc-uk.org
Helpline: 020 7631 0285

Association of Breastfeeding Mothers
Support and information from qualified breastfeeding counsellors.
Website: http://abm.me.uk
Helpline: 08444 122 949

Birth Trauma Association
Offers support to women struggling to handle the event of childbirth.
Website: www.birthtraumaassociation.org.uk

Bliss
Helps families whose babies are born prematurely.
Website: www.bliss.org.uk
Helpline: 0500 618 140

Cry-Sis
An organisation that offers support for parents with excessively crying, sleepless and demanding babies.
Website: www.cry-sis.org.uk
Helpline: 0845 228 669

Depression Alliance
Help for all kinds of depression, including post-natal depression.
Website: www.depressionalliance.org
Telephone: 0845 123 2320

Direct.gov

The Government's website for public services. Find out here about benefits and maternity/paternity allowances, childcare, Sure Start Children's Centres and lots more.
Website: www.direct.gov.uk

Family and Parenting Institute

Information and guidance from experts in the field. Also runs the Family Friendly scheme, who have their own website: www.wearefamilyfriendly.org/family/home
Website: www.familyandparenting.org

Family Information Service

Advice, information and support for parents of children with any kind of disability.
Website: www.cafamily.org.uk
Helpline: 0808 808 3555

Family Lives

Provides help and support in all aspects of family life, and runs the telephone advice service Parentline.
Website: http://familylives.org.uk
Helpline: 0808 800 2222

Fatherhood Institute

A national organisation working to ensure a positive relationship between children and their fathers.
Website: www.fatherhoodinstitute.org
Telephone: 0845 634 1328

Foundation for the Study of Infant Deaths

Dedicated to researching the causes of sudden infant death, and supporting affected families.
Website: http://fsid.org.uk
Helpline: 0808 802 6868

Gingerbread
An organisation dedicated to helping single parents.
Website: www.gingerbread.org.uk
Helpline: 0808 802 0925

Home Start
Supports parents with young children under the age of five.
Website: www.home-start.org.uk
Telephone: 0800 068 63 68

HomeDad
Puts stay-at-home dads in touch with one another, and offers information and guidance.
Website: http://homedad.org.uk

La Leche League
Support for breastfeeding.
Website: www.laleche.org.uk
Helpline: 0845 120 2918

Meet-a-Mum Association
Works to bring mums together for companionship and support.
Website: www.mama.bm

Miscarriage Association
Offers support for anyone affected by miscarriage, ectopic pregnancy or molar pregnancy.
Website: www.miscarriageassociation.org.uk
Helpline: 01924 200 799

National Childbirth Trust (NCT)
Support from pregnancy through to parenthood at national and local levels.
Website: www.nct.org.uk
Helpline: 08457 90 90 90

Perinatal Illness UK
Support for people affected by antenatal depression, postnatal depression and birth trauma.
Website: www.pni-uk.com

PNI ORG UK
Online information and support for women affected by post-natal depression.
Website: www.pni.org.uk

Relate
Provides relationship information and counselling for couples.
Website: www.relate.org.uk
Telephone: 0300 100 1234

Samaritans
Support for anyone who's struggling to cope.
Website: www.samaritans.org
Helpline: 0300 330 0700

SANDS (Stillbirth and Neonatal Death Charity)
Offering support for anyone affected by the death of a baby.
Website: www.uk-sands.org
Helpline: 020 7436 5881

The Child Bereavement Trust
Support for families touched by child bereavement.
Website: www.childbereavement.org.uk
Helpline: 01494 568900

Tommy's
Works to prevent miscarriage, premature birth and stillbirth.
Website: www.tommys.org
Helpline: 0800 0147 800

Twins and Multiple Births Association
Support and information for parents of twins, triplets and more.
Website: www.tamba.org.uk
Helpline: 0800 138 0509

What About the Children?
An organisation that works to inform people about the emotional needs of children under three years of age.
Website: www.whataboutthechildren.org.uk
Telephone: 0845 602 7145

Working Families
Works to help parents who work achieve a good work–life balance.
Website: www.workingfamilies.org.uk

USEFUL WEBSITES
The following websites contain a wealth of information on pregnancy, birth, babies, toddlers, children and parenting:

Ask Moxie: www.askmoxie.org
Baby Centre: www.babycentre.co.uk
Baby Expert: www.babyexpert.com
Baby World: www.babyworld.co.uk
BBC: www.bbc.co.uk/parenting
Boots Parenting Club: www.boots.com/en/Mother-
    Baby/Parenting-Club
Bounty: www.bounty.com/baby
Emma's Diary: www.emmasdiary.co.uk
Family and Parenting: www.familyandparenting.co.uk
iVillage: www.ivillage.co.uk/channel/parenting
Mumsnet: www.mumsnet.com
Netmums: www.netmums.com
Positive Parenting: www.parenting.org.uk
Pregnancy.co.uk: www.pregnancy.co.uk

MOVIES

I went through a phase while pregnant of watching films about babies and pregnancy (actually, at one point, a week before I gave birth, it extended to watching births on nature programmes, until a particularly graphic rhino birth turned me green!). If you're in the mood for a dose of babydom, one of the following may take your fancy:

Juno (2007)
My personal favourite – a witty, quirky, lovely film.

Knocked Up (2007)
Hilarious, edgy and true to life, without a whiff of cheese.

Life as We Know It (2010)
I love this film – funny and touching in equal measure.

Waitress (2007)
Keri Russell stars in this award-winning feel-good film.

Using my husband (who hates chick flicks) as a benchmark, I reckon these are films for both mums and dads. But if you're an ardent girly film fan, and you don't mind a good dose of cheese, you could also revisit some old classics: *Father of the Bride* (1995), *Jack and Sarah* (1995), *Junior* (1994), *Look Who's Talking* (1989), *Look Who's Talking Too* (1990), *Three Men and a Baby* (1987) and *Nine Months* (1995) (don't make my mistake and confuse this with the film *Nine and a Half Weeks* – though Dad might enjoy that one a little more!).

Index

Lightning Source UK Ltd.
Milton Keynes UK
UKOW04f1023250215

246876UK00001B/5/P